CARNIVORE DIET

A Unique Dive into Carnivore Living –

Unveiling Tantalizing Tastes and Nutritional

Wisdom with tens of new recipes where Each

Bite Unlocks a Symphony of Health and

Flavor

COLE TAYLOR

TABLE OF CONTENTS

Introduction

Welcome to the world of the Carnivore Diet—a lifestyle choice that challenges conventional wisdom, invites you to reevaluate your relationship with food, and promises a journey of unparalleled health and vitality. In this book, we embark on a fascinating exploration into the depths of carnivore living, where each bite unlocks not only a symphony of flavor but also a wealth of nutritional wisdom.

The Carnivore Diet, often considered a radical departure from mainstream dietary advice, is rooted in the fundamental principle of consuming animal products exclusively. It's a diet that harks back to our primal instincts, drawing inspiration from our hunter-gatherer ancestors who thrived on animal foods for millennia. But beyond its evolutionary underpinnings, the Carnivore Diet represents a bold departure from the complex world of modern nutrition—a return to simplicity, purity, and the unadulterated nourishment found in nature's bounty.

In this book, we delve deep into the science behind the Carnivore Diet, dispelling myths and misconceptions while uncovering the profound health benefits that await those who dare to embrace this carnivorous lifestyle. We explore the nutritional foundations of the diet, from the essential role of protein and fat to the importance of micronutrients in promoting optimal health and well-being. And we confront the skeptics head-on, addressing concerns and potential risks with evidence-based insights and practical guidance.

But the Carnivore Diet is more than just a nutritional regimen—it's a way of life. And in these pages, we guide you through every aspect of that lifestyle, from preparing delicious and nutritious meals to navigating social situations with confidence and grace. We provide you with the tools and techniques you need to succeed on your carnivore journey, whether you're a seasoned pro or a curious newcomer eager to explore new culinary horizons.

Throughout this book, you'll find a treasure trove of tantalizing recipes, each one carefully crafted to showcase the diverse flavors and textures of the carnivore diet. From hearty breakfasts to elegant dinners, from savory snacks to mouthwatering desserts, we invite you to savor the rich tapestry of tastes that await you in the world of carnivore cuisine.

But perhaps most importantly, this book is a celebration of the transformative power of the Carnivore Diet—a testament to the countless individuals who have reclaimed their health, vitality, and zest for life through the simple act of eating like a carnivore. Their stories inspire us, their journeys inspire us, and their successes remind us that the path to optimal health is as individual as we are.

So join us now as we embark on this extraordinary journey into the heart of carnivore living. Whether you're seeking to improve your health, enhance your performance, or simply explore new culinary horizons, the Carnivore Diet offers a world of possibilities waiting to be discovered. And with each page you turn, each recipe you try, and each bite you savor, you'll be one step closer to unlocking the boundless potential of the carnivore lifestyle. Welcome aboard.

Chapter 1

Introduction to Carnivore Living

Defining the Carnivore Diet

The Carnivore Diet has surged in popularity in recent years, capturing the attention of health enthusiasts, fitness communities, and individuals seeking radical dietary approaches. Rooted in the premise of consuming exclusively animal-based foods while eliminating plant-derived products, the Carnivore Diet has sparked debates, controversies, and fervent advocacy. In this comprehensive discourse, we delve into the nuances, controversies, potential benefits, and risks associated with the Carnivore Diet.

- **Origins and Evolution**

The Carnivore Diet finds its roots in historical accounts of indigenous societies and early human ancestors, whose diets primarily consisted of animal products due to environmental constraints and limited access to vegetation. However, the modern incarnation of the Carnivore Diet gained momentum in the 20th century, particularly with the works of controversial figures like Vilhjalmur Stefansson, a Canadian Arctic explorer who famously lived for prolonged periods on an all-meat diet without apparent ill effects. Stefansson's experiences and subsequent studies contributed to the revival of interest in carnivorous eating patterns.

- **Defining the Carnivore Diet**

At its core, the Carnivore Diet is characterized by its strict adherence to animal-derived foods, typically including meat, fish, eggs, and certain dairy products while eschewing plant-based foods such as fruits, vegetables, grains, legumes, and nuts. Proponents of the Carnivore Diet often emphasize the consumption of fatty cuts of meat, organs, and bone marrow, touting the nutritional completeness and bioavailability of nutrients inherent in animal-based foods.

- **Nutritional Composition and Controversies**

The nutritional composition of the Carnivore Diet is notably high in protein and fat while lacking in carbohydrates, fiber, and many essential vitamins and minerals commonly found in plant foods. While advocates assert that animal products provide all necessary nutrients in optimal forms, critics raise concerns about potential deficiencies, particularly in vitamins C, E, and K, as well as fiber and various phytonutrients crucial for health.

- **Physiological Mechanisms and Alleged Benefits**

Proponents of the Carnivore Diet often cite various physiological mechanisms and alleged benefits associated with its adoption. These include:

> **Improved metabolic health:** Advocates claim that eliminating carbohydrates can lead to better blood sugar control, reduced insulin resistance, and enhanced fat metabolism, potentially benefiting individuals with conditions like type 2 diabetes and obesity.

> **Gut health:** Some proponents argue that eliminating plant foods can alleviate digestive issues such as bloating, gas, and irritable bowel syndrome (IBS), although scientific evidence supporting this claim remains limited and inconclusive.

➢ **Autoimmune conditions:** Anecdotal reports suggest that the Carnivore Diet may alleviate symptoms of autoimmune disorders like rheumatoid arthritis, psoriasis, and inflammatory bowel disease (IBD), although rigorous clinical trials are lacking.

- **Controversies and Criticisms**

  Despite its growing popularity, the Carnivore Diet remains highly controversial, drawing criticisms from various quarters:

➢ **Nutritional deficiencies:** Skeptics warn that the exclusion of plant foods can lead to deficiencies in essential nutrients like fiber, vitamins, minerals, and phytonutrients, potentially increasing the risk of long-term health complications.

➢ **Sustainability:** Critics argue that promoting a diet heavily reliant on animal agriculture is environmentally unsustainable, contributing to deforestation, greenhouse gas emissions, and animal welfare concerns.

➢ **Long-term health effects:** The long-term health implications of the Carnivore Diet remain uncertain, with limited scientific evidence available to assess its safety and efficacy over extended periods.

- **Clinical Evidence and Research Gaps**

  While anecdotal reports and small-scale studies have documented various outcomes associated with the Carnivore Diet, robust clinical evidence remains scarce. Most existing research suffers from methodological limitations, including small sample sizes, short duration, lack of control groups, and reliance on self-reported data. Additionally, ethical considerations and practical challenges often hinder the conduct of rigorous, long-term trials examining the Carnivore Diet's effects on health outcomes.

- **Individual Variability and Personalization**

  An important aspect often overlooked in discussions about the Carnivore Diet is the concept of individual variability and dietary personalization. While some individuals may thrive on a predominantly animal-based diet, others may experience adverse effects or struggle to meet their nutritional needs without plant foods. Factors such as genetics, microbiome composition, metabolic health, activity level, and food preferences can profoundly influence an individual's response to dietary interventions, highlighting the need for personalized approaches to nutrition.

The Carnivore Diet represents a radical departure from conventional dietary recommendations, emphasizing the exclusive consumption of animal-based foods while excluding plant-derived products. While some individuals report benefits such as weight loss, improved energy levels, and symptom relief from various health conditions, the scientific evidence supporting the Carnivore Diet's safety and efficacy remains limited and inconclusive. As such, individuals considering embarking on the Carnivore Diet should approach it with caution, seeking guidance from qualified healthcare professionals and considering potential long-term implications for health, sustainability, and ethical considerations. Moreover, acknowledging the diverse responses to dietary interventions underscores the importance of personalized nutrition strategies tailored to individual needs, preferences, and health goals. Ultimately, navigating the Carnivore Diet landscape requires a balanced evaluation of available evidence, careful consideration of ethical and environmental implications, and a commitment to prioritize long-term health and well-being.

Historical Context: Origins and Evolution

The Carnivore Diet, a dietary regimen emphasizing the consumption of animal-derived foods while excluding plant-based products, has gained traction in recent years, captivating the interest of health enthusiasts, fitness communities, and individuals seeking alternative approaches to nutrition. To understand the Carnivore Diet fully, it's essential to explore its historical origins and evolution, tracing its development from early human dietary patterns to its modern incarnation. In this comprehensive discussion, we delve into the historical context of the Carnivore Diet, examining its roots, influences, and evolutionary trajectory.

- **Ancestral Diets: Prehistoric Foundations**

The origins of the Carnivore Diet can be traced back to our prehistoric ancestors, whose dietary patterns were shaped by environmental factors, geographic locations, and evolutionary adaptations. Early humans were hunter-gatherers, relying on a diverse array of foods obtained through hunting, fishing, and foraging. While plant foods undoubtedly played a significant role in ancestral diets, particularly during periods of abundance, archaeological evidence suggests that animal products comprised a substantial portion of prehistoric human nutrition, especially in regions where plant resources were scarce or seasonal.

- **Paleolithic Perspectives: Hunter-Gatherer Insights**

The Paleolithic era, often referred to as the Stone Age, spans from approximately 2.6 million years ago to around 10,000 years ago. During this period, humans subsisted on diets primarily composed of wild game, fish, shellfish, and occasionally gathered plant foods such as fruits, roots, and tubers. Research examining Paleolithic dietary patterns provides insights into the nutritional composition and ecological context of ancestral diets, highlighting the prominence of animal foods and the adaptive advantages conferred by high-protein, nutrient-dense diets in challenging environments.

- **Ethnographic Evidence: Indigenous Traditions and Practices**

Ethnographic studies of contemporary hunter-gatherer societies offer valuable insights into traditional dietary practices and cultural attitudes toward animal foods. Many indigenous populations, such as the Inuit of the Arctic, the Maasai of East Africa, and the Mongolian nomads of the Central Asian steppes, have subsisted for generations on diets predominantly composed of animal products, including meat, fish, organs, and animal fats. These societies exemplify the nutritional adequacy and metabolic adaptability of animal-based diets in diverse ecological settings, challenging conventional notions of dietary diversity and plant-centric nutrition.

- **Historical Anecdotes: Explorers, Adventurers, and Pioneers**

The Carnivore Diet's modern resurgence can be attributed in part to historical anecdotes, accounts, and observations of explorers, adventurers, and pioneers who documented their experiences with meat-centric diets. One such figure is Vilhjalmur Stefansson, a Canadian Arctic explorer who, along with his colleague Karsten Anderson, lived for extended periods among the Inuit and subsisted primarily on a diet of meat, fish, and animal fats. Stefansson's expeditions and subsequent writings, including "Not by Bread

Alone" and "The Fat of the Land," challenged prevailing dietary dogmas and sparked renewed interest in carnivorous eating patterns.

- **Medical Context: Therapeutic Applications and Clinical Experiments**

  Throughout history, physicians, scientists, and researchers have explored the therapeutic potential of animal-based diets for treating various medical conditions and metabolic disorders. In the early 20th century, pioneering physicians such as Dr. Blake F. Donaldson advocated for low-carbohydrate, high-fat diets as therapeutic interventions for obesity, diabetes, and cardiovascular disease, drawing inspiration from his observations of traditional

Inuit diets and clinical experiences treating patients with metabolic syndrome.

- **Contemporary Influences: Scientific Advances and Cultural Shifts**

The contemporary resurgence of interest in the Carnivore Diet can be attributed to a confluence of factors, including advancements in nutritional science, popularization of low-carbohydrate dietary approaches, and cultural shifts toward ancestral health movements and alternative lifestyles. The emergence of the internet and social media platforms has facilitated the dissemination of information, testimonials, and personal anecdotes from individuals experimenting with carnivorous eating patterns, fostering a vibrant online community of Carnivore Diet enthusiasts and advocates.

The Carnivore Diet's historical context provides valuable insights into the evolutionary foundations, cultural practices, and scientific underpinnings of animal-based eating patterns. From prehistoric hunter-gatherers to contemporary proponents, the Carnivore Diet reflects a continuum of dietary traditions, beliefs, and adaptations shaped by human evolution, ecological pressures, and cultural preferences. While the modern Carnivore Diet may diverge from ancestral diets in certain respects, its resurgence underscores a broader reevaluation of dietary paradigms, nutritional dogmas, and individualized approaches to health and wellness. By navigating the historical landscape of the Carnivore Diet with an open mind and critical perspective, we can gain a deeper appreciation for its complexities, controversies, and potential implications for human health and nutrition in the modern world.

Why Carnivore? Exploring the Benefits

Exploring the benefits of the Carnivore Diet entails a comprehensive examination of its potential physiological effects, purported advantages, and reported outcomes. Despite its controversial nature and departure from conventional dietary recommendations, proponents of the Carnivore Diet advocate for its adoption based on various perceived benefits, ranging from improved metabolic health and weight management to enhanced mental clarity and athletic performance. In this discussion, we delve into the reasons why individuals may choose to embrace the Carnivore Diet, exploring the scientific evidence, anecdotal reports, and theoretical mechanisms underlying its purported benefits.

- **Metabolic Health and Insulin Sensitivity**

  One of the primary reasons individuals turn to the Carnivore Diet is its potential to improve metabolic health and insulin sensitivity. By eliminating carbohydrates and minimizing fluctuations in blood sugar levels, the Carnivore Diet may help regulate insulin secretion and reduce insulin resistance, thereby mitigating the risk of metabolic disorders such as type 2 diabetes and obesity. Some studies suggest that low-carbohydrate diets can lead to favorable changes in metabolic biomarkers, including improved glycemic control, reduced triglycerides, and increased HDL cholesterol levels, although long-term effects on cardiovascular health remain debated.

- **Weight Loss and Body Composition**

Weight loss and body composition changes are common motivations for adopting the Carnivore Diet, with many individuals reporting significant reductions in body fat, increased lean muscle mass, and improvements in overall body composition. The high-protein, satiating nature of animal-based foods may promote feelings of fullness and satiety, leading to spontaneous caloric restriction and enhanced fat metabolism. Moreover, the absence of carbohydrates may facilitate ketosis, a metabolic state characterized by the utilization of fat for energy, which can accelerate fat loss and promote weight maintenance over time.

- **Digestive Health and Gut Function**

Another purported benefit of the Carnivore Diet is its potential to alleviate digestive issues and improve gut function in susceptible individuals. By eliminating plant foods and their associated anti-nutrients, fibers, and fermentable carbohydrates, some individuals report reductions in bloating, gas, diarrhea, and other gastrointestinal symptoms commonly associated with conditions like irritable bowel syndrome (IBS) and inflammatory bowel disease (IBD). However, the scientific evidence supporting these claims remains limited, and individual responses to dietary interventions can vary widely.

- **Autoimmune Conditions and Inflammation**

Anecdotal reports and emerging research suggest that the Carnivore Diet may have therapeutic implications for individuals with autoimmune conditions characterized by chronic inflammation and immune dysregulation. By removing potential dietary triggers, such as lectins, phytates, and other plant-derived compounds, the Carnivore Diet may alleviate symptoms associated with autoimmune disorders such as rheumatoid arthritis, psoriasis, and inflammatory bowel disease. However, controlled clinical trials are needed to validate these observations and elucidate the underlying mechanisms of action.

- **Mental Clarity and Cognitive Function**

  Some proponents of the Carnivore Diet claim improvements in mental clarity, cognitive function, and mood stability as additional benefits of eliminating carbohydrates and optimizing nutrient intake. While the scientific evidence supporting these assertions is largely anecdotal and subjective, proponents suggest that stable blood sugar levels, increased ketone production, and enhanced neurotransmitter synthesis may contribute to improved mental acuity, focus, and mood regulation. However, individual responses to dietary interventions can vary, and more research is needed to elucidate the relationship between diet and brain health.

- **Athletic Performance and Recovery**

  Athletes and fitness enthusiasts may be drawn to the Carnivore Diet for its potential to enhance athletic performance, recovery, and muscle protein synthesis. Animal-based foods are rich sources of high-quality protein, essential amino acids, and bioavailable nutrients necessary for muscle repair, growth, and recovery following intense exercise. Moreover, the anti-inflammatory properties of animal fats and omega-3 fatty acids may help mitigate exercise-induced inflammation and oxidative stress, potentially improving recovery times and exercise tolerance.

- **Simplified Eating Patterns and Food Choices**

From a practical standpoint, the simplicity and convenience of the Carnivore Diet appeal to individuals seeking to streamline their eating patterns and food choices. By focusing exclusively on animal-derived foods and eliminating complex meal planning, food preparation, and dietary restrictions associated with plant-based diets, the Carnivore Diet offers a straightforward approach to nutrition that resonates with some individuals. Moreover, the satiating nature of animal fats and proteins may reduce cravings, hunger, and the temptation to indulge in processed or hyperpalatable foods.

The Carnivore Diet offers a compelling yet controversial approach to nutrition, with proponents touting various potential benefits ranging from improved metabolic health and weight management to enhanced mental clarity and athletic performance. While anecdotal reports and emerging research suggest promising outcomes associated with the Carnivore Diet, the scientific evidence supporting its efficacy, safety, and long-term sustainability remains limited and inconclusive.

As such, individuals considering embarking on the Carnivore Diet should approach it with caution, seeking guidance from qualified healthcare professionals and considering potential risks, individual variability, and ethical considerations. By navigating the potential benefits of the Carnivore Diet with an open mind and critical perspective, we can gain a deeper understanding of its complexities, controversies, and implications for human health and well-being.

Chapter 2

Understanding the Science Behind Carnivore Nutrition

Nutritional Foundations: Protein, Fat, and Micronutrients

The carnivore diet, a dietary approach primarily consisting of animal-derived foods, has garnered attention in recent years for its purported health benefits and controversial nature. Advocates of the carnivore diet argue that it can improve various health markers, including weight loss, metabolic health, and mental clarity. However, critics express concerns about potential nutrient deficiencies and long-term health implications. This section aims to explore the nutritional foundations of the carnivore diet, focusing on its key components: protein, fat, and micronutrients.

- **Protein**

Protein serves as a fundamental building block for the human body, playing essential roles in muscle repair, hormone synthesis, and immune function. In the context of the carnivore diet, protein takes center stage, as animal-derived foods are the primary source of this macronutrient. Meat, fish, poultry, and eggs are rich sources of complete protein, containing all essential amino acids necessary for human health.

One of the primary arguments in favor of the carnivore diet is its ability to provide high-quality, bioavailable protein. Unlike plant-based proteins, which may lack certain essential amino acids or contain anti-nutrients that inhibit absorption, animal proteins are easily digestible and contain optimal ratios of amino acids. This ensures that individuals following the carnivore diet can meet their protein needs without resorting to supplementation or careful food combining.

Moreover, the protein content of animal foods can vary, allowing individuals to tailor their intake based on their activity levels, muscle mass, and health goals. For example, athletes or individuals seeking muscle growth may benefit from higher protein intake, while sedentary individuals may require less. The carnivore diet provides flexibility in protein consumption, allowing individuals to adjust their intake based on individual needs.

- **Fat**

Fat is another crucial component of the carnivore diet, providing energy, insulation, and serving as a precursor for hormone production. Animal fats, such as those found in meat, poultry, fish, and eggs, are rich in saturated and monounsaturated fats, which have been unfairly demonized in the past but are now recognized as important for overall health.

Contrary to popular belief, saturated fats do not necessarily contribute to heart disease when consumed as part of a balanced diet. In fact, they play vital roles in cellular membrane structure, hormone regulation, and the absorption of fat-soluble vitamins. By embracing animal fats as a primary energy source, individuals following the carnivore diet can achieve satiety, stabilize blood sugar levels, and promote metabolic flexibility.

Additionally, the inclusion of omega-3 fatty acids from fatty fish such as salmon, mackerel, and sardines further enhances the nutritional profile of the carnivore diet. Omega-3s are renowned for their anti-inflammatory properties and cardiovascular benefits, making them an essential component of a healthy dietary pattern.

- **Micronutrients**

While the carnivore diet prioritizes animal-derived foods, concerns regarding micronutrient adequacy have been raised due to the exclusion of plant foods. Plants are rich sources of vitamins, minerals, antioxidants, and phytonutrients, which play critical roles in supporting overall health and reducing the risk of chronic disease.

However, proponents of the carnivore diet argue that animal foods contain an abundance of essential micronutrients in highly bioavailable forms. Meat, for example, is an excellent source of B vitamins, including B12, which is primarily found in animal products and crucial for nerve function and red blood cell formation. Additionally, organ meats such as liver are nutrient powerhouses, providing concentrated amounts of vitamins A, D, E, and K, as well as minerals like iron, zinc, and selenium.

Furthermore, the carnivore diet emphasizes the consumption of nose-to-tail animal products, ensuring that individuals obtain a wide array of micronutrients. While plant foods may offer certain micronutrients in higher quantities, the carnivore diet argues for the efficiency and bioavailability of animal-derived sources, which can meet or exceed nutritional requirements.

Critics of the carnivore diet often express concerns about potential deficiencies in vitamin C and fiber, which are commonly associated with plant foods. However, proponents argue that vitamin C requirements may decrease on a low-carbohydrate, ketogenic diet due to reduced glucose competition for vitamin C uptake in cells. Additionally, fiber, while important for gut health, may not be essential for everyone and can be obtained through supplementation if necessary.

The carnivore diet represents a dietary approach centered around animal-derived foods, prioritizing protein, fat, and micronutrients while excluding plant foods. Proponents argue that the carnivore diet offers numerous health benefits, including improved metabolic health, weight loss, and mental clarity. However, concerns regarding long-term sustainability and potential nutrient deficiencies remain topics of debate.

The nutritional foundations of the carnivore diet highlight the importance of high-quality protein, healthy fats, and nutrient-dense animal products in supporting overall health and well-being. While further research is needed to fully understand the long-term implications of the carnivore diet, individuals should prioritize nutrient adequacy, listen to their bodies, and consult with healthcare professionals before making significant dietary changes. Ultimately, the carnivore diet represents one approach to nutrition among many, and its suitability may vary depending on individual needs, preferences, and health goals.

Debunking Myths and Misconceptions

The carnivore diet has gained significant attention in recent years as a controversial dietary approach centered around the exclusive consumption of animal-derived foods. Despite its growing popularity, the carnivore diet is often shrouded in myths and misconceptions, leading to skepticism and criticism from both the general public and the scientific community. This part aims to debunk common myths and misconceptions surrounding the carnivore diet, providing a nuanced perspective based on scientific evidence and expert opinion.

- **Myth 1: The Carnivore Diet Lacks Essential Nutrients**

One of the most prevalent myths about the carnivore diet is that it leads to nutrient deficiencies due to the exclusion of plant-based foods. Critics argue that plants are rich sources of vitamins, minerals, and antioxidants, essential for maintaining overall health and preventing chronic disease.

However, proponents of the carnivore diet assert that animal-derived foods contain all the essential nutrients necessary for human health in highly bioavailable forms. Meat, fish, poultry, and eggs are rich sources of protein, essential amino acids, vitamins (such as B vitamins and fat-soluble vitamins), minerals (including iron, zinc, and selenium), and healthy fats. Furthermore, organ meats such as liver provide concentrated amounts of micronutrients, often surpassing those found in plant foods.

While it is true that some plant foods offer unique phytonutrients and fiber, proponents argue that these nutrients are not essential and can be obtained through animal sources or supplementation if necessary. Additionally, the carnivore diet emphasizes nose-to-tail eating, ensuring a diverse array of nutrients from different animal parts.

Research on the nutritional adequacy of the carnivore diet is limited but suggests that individuals can thrive on this dietary pattern when properly planned and executed. However, further studies are needed to better understand the long-term implications of the carnivore diet on nutrient status and overall health.

- **Myth 2: The Carnivore Diet Causes Heart Disease and Increases Cholesterol Levels**

Another common myth surrounding the carnivore diet is that it promotes heart disease and elevates cholesterol levels due to its high intake of saturated fats and cholesterol-containing foods.

Historically, saturated fats and dietary cholesterol have been vilified as major contributors to heart disease based on observational studies and outdated dietary guidelines. However, more recent research has challenged this paradigm, suggesting that the relationship between dietary fat, cholesterol, and heart health is more complex than previously thought.

Studies have shown that saturated fats from animal sources may not have the detrimental effects on cholesterol levels and cardiovascular health once believed. In fact, some evidence suggests that replacing saturated fats with refined carbohydrates may increase the risk of heart disease, while saturated fats may improve lipid profiles and insulin sensitivity.

Furthermore, cholesterol levels are influenced by various factors, including genetics, lifestyle, and overall dietary pattern. While some individuals may experience an increase in cholesterol levels initially when transitioning to the carnivore diet, it is not necessarily indicative of poor cardiovascular health. Moreover, not all cholesterol is created equal, and the ratio of LDL to HDL cholesterol, as well as particle size and density, may be more relevant indicators of cardiovascular risk.

Proponents of the carnivore diet argue that the consumption of animal fats and proteins can support cardiovascular health by promoting satiety, reducing inflammation, and improving metabolic function. Additionally, the exclusion of processed foods, refined carbohydrates, and vegetable oils may contribute to better heart health outcomes.

However, individuals with pre-existing cardiovascular conditions or concerns should consult with healthcare professionals before adopting the carnivore diet and monitor their health markers regularly.

- **Myth 3: The Carnivore Diet Is Unhealthy and Unsustainable**

Critics often characterize the carnivore diet as unhealthy and unsustainable, citing concerns about its environmental impact, ethical implications, and long-term health consequences.

From an environmental perspective, the carnivore diet has been criticized for its reliance on animal agriculture, which is associated with greenhouse gas emissions, deforestation, and water usage. Critics argue that promoting the consumption of animal products exacerbates environmental degradation and contributes to climate change.

While it is true that animal agriculture has significant environmental consequences, proponents of the carnivore diet argue that regenerative farming practices, such as rotational grazing and holistic land management, can mitigate these impacts. By supporting local, sustainable farmers who prioritize animal welfare and environmental stewardship, individuals following the carnivore diet can minimize their ecological footprint.

From an ethical standpoint, concerns are raised about the treatment of animals raised for food and the moral implications of consuming animal products. While factory farming practices are indeed problematic and raise valid ethical concerns, proponents of the carnivore diet advocate for the consumption of ethically sourced, pasture-raised animal products from farms that prioritize animal welfare and humane treatment.

Additionally, critics argue that the carnivore diet is unsustainable in the long term and may lead to nutrient deficiencies, gastrointestinal issues, and other health problems. However, anecdotal evidence and clinical experience suggest that many individuals thrive on the carnivore diet, experiencing improvements in various health markers, including weight loss, metabolic health, and mental well-being.

While the carnivore diet may not be suitable for everyone and requires careful planning and monitoring, proponents argue that it can be a viable and sustainable dietary approach for certain individuals, particularly those with specific health conditions or dietary preferences.

The carnivore diet is a controversial dietary approach that is often misunderstood and misrepresented. By debunking common myths and misconceptions surrounding the carnivore diet, we can gain a more nuanced understanding of its potential benefits and limitations.

While the carnivore diet may not be suitable for everyone and raises valid concerns about nutrient adequacy, environmental impact, and ethical considerations, it is essential to evaluate the scientific evidence and individual experiences objectively. Further research is needed to better understand the long-term implications of the carnivore diet on health, including its effects on nutrient status, cardiovascular health, and sustainability.

Ultimately, individuals should approach the carnivore diet with caution, consult with healthcare professionals, and make informed decisions based on their unique needs, preferences, and ethical considerations. By fostering open dialogue and critical thinking, we can continue to explore the potential of the carnivore diet while addressing legitimate concerns and promoting overall health and well-being.

Health Impacts and Potential Risks

Proponents of the carnivore diet advocate for its potential to improve weight loss, metabolic health, and mental clarity. However, concerns have been raised regarding the health impacts and potential risks associated with this extreme dietary pattern. This part aims to explore the health impacts and potential risks of the carnivore diet, considering both its physiological effects and broader implications for long-term health and well-being.

- **Physiological Impacts**

➢ **Nutrient Adequacy**

One of the primary concerns regarding the carnivore diet is its potential to lead to nutrient deficiencies due to the exclusion of plant-based foods. While animal-derived foods contain essential nutrients such as protein, fat, vitamins, and minerals, the absence of fruits, vegetables, grains, and legumes may result in inadequate intake of certain micronutrients, fiber, and phytonutrients.

Vitamin C, for example, is predominantly found in plant foods and plays a critical role in immune function, collagen synthesis, and antioxidant defense. While some proponents argue that vitamin C requirements may decrease on a low-carbohydrate, ketogenic diet due to reduced glucose competition for vitamin C uptake in cells, individuals following the carnivore diet may still be at risk of deficiency if they do not consume sufficient quantities of organ meats or supplement with vitamin C.

Additionally, fiber is essential for digestive health, bowel regularity, and the prevention of chronic diseases such as colorectal cancer and cardiovascular disease. While proponents of the carnivore diet argue that fiber is not essential and may even be detrimental to gut health in some cases, the long-term consequences of fiber restriction on digestive function and overall health remain unclear.

➢ **Gut Microbiota**

Another area of concern is the potential impact of the carnivore diet on gut microbiota composition and diversity. Plant-based foods are rich sources of dietary fiber, prebiotics, and polyphenols, which support the growth and diversity of beneficial gut bacteria. By contrast, the carnivore diet restricts these fermentable substrates, potentially leading to dysbiosis, gut inflammation, and impaired gut barrier function.

Emerging research suggests that alterations in gut microbiota composition and function are associated with various health conditions, including obesity, metabolic syndrome, autoimmune diseases, and mental health disorders. While anecdotal reports suggest that some individuals experience improvements in digestive symptoms and autoimmune conditions on the carnivore diet, the long-term effects on gut health and microbiota remain uncertain.

> **Metabolic Health**

Proponents of the carnivore diet often claim improvements in metabolic health, including weight loss, blood sugar regulation, and lipid profiles. By eliminating carbohydrates and processed foods, the carnivore diet may induce ketosis, a metabolic state characterized by the production of ketone bodies from fat metabolism.

Ketosis has been associated with various health benefits, including appetite suppression, enhanced fat oxidation, and improved insulin sensitivity. However, the carnivore diet's high intake of saturated fats and cholesterol-containing foods may raise concerns about cardiovascular health, particularly in individuals predisposed to hypercholesterolemia or heart disease.

Furthermore, the long-term effects of sustained ketosis on metabolic health, hormone regulation, and organ function are not well understood. While short-term studies suggest potential benefits, more research is needed to evaluate the safety and efficacy of the carnivore diet for long-term weight management and metabolic health.

- **Potential Risks**

➢ **Nutrient Deficiencies**

As previously mentioned, the carnivore diet may increase the risk of nutrient deficiencies, particularly in vitamins and minerals that are primarily found in plant-based foods. While animal-derived foods provide essential nutrients, they may not always meet recommended dietary intakes for certain micronutrients, such as vitamin C, folate, magnesium, and potassium.

Deficiencies in these nutrients can lead to a range of health problems, including immune dysfunction, anemia, cardiovascular disease, and bone disorders. Individuals following the carnivore diet should be vigilant about meeting their nutritional needs through a variety of animal foods, including organ meats, seafood, eggs, and dairy, as well as supplementation if necessary.

➢ **Gastrointestinal Issues**

Some individuals may experience gastrointestinal issues when transitioning to the carnivore diet, including constipation, diarrhea, bloating, and abdominal discomfort. These symptoms may be attributed to changes in gut microbiota composition, fiber restriction, and alterations in bowel habits.

While proponents argue that these symptoms are temporary and resolve over time as the body adapts to the carnivore diet, others may experience persistent digestive problems that impact their quality of life. It is essential to listen to your body, make gradual dietary changes, and seek guidance from healthcare professionals if you experience severe or prolonged gastrointestinal issues on the carnivore diet.

➢ **Psychological and Social Impacts**

In addition to physiological risks, the carnivore diet may have psychological and social implications for individuals' mental health and well-being. The restrictive nature of the diet, which excludes entire food groups and limits food choices to animal-derived foods, can lead to feelings of isolation, deprivation, and disordered eating behaviors.

Moreover, adhering to the carnivore diet may pose challenges in social settings, where plant-based options are limited, and dietary restrictions may conflict with cultural or social norms. Individuals following the carnivore diet should be mindful of their emotional relationship with food, seek support from peers and healthcare professionals, and prioritize balance, flexibility, and enjoyment in their dietary choices.

The carnivore diet represents a controversial dietary approach characterized by the exclusive consumption of animal-derived foods. While proponents tout potential health benefits, including weight loss, metabolic improvements, and mental clarity, concerns have been raised regarding its potential health impacts and risks.

Physiologically, the carnivore diet may increase the risk of nutrient deficiencies, gut microbiota dysbiosis, and metabolic disturbances. Nutrient adequacy, particularly in vitamins and minerals primarily found in plant-based foods, is a significant concern, as is the potential impact on gastrointestinal health and digestive function.

Furthermore, the carnivore diet may have psychological and social implications, including feelings of isolation, deprivation, and disordered eating behaviors. Individuals considering the carnivore diet should carefully weigh the potential benefits and risks, seek guidance from healthcare professionals, and prioritize a balanced and sustainable approach to nutrition and overall health.

Further research is needed to better understand the long-term effects of the carnivore diet on health outcomes, including its impact on nutrient status, metabolic health, gut microbiota, and psychological well-being. In the meantime, individuals should approach the carnivore diet with caution, listen to their bodies, and make informed decisions based on their unique needs, preferences, and health goals.

Chapter 3

Preparing for the Carnivore Lifestyle

Transitioning from Other Diets

Transitioning to a carnivore diet from other dietary patterns can be a significant change for many individuals. Whether coming from a standard Western diet rich in carbohydrates, a plant-based diet, or any other eating regimen, this shift requires careful consideration and planning to ensure optimal health and well-being. In this part, we will explore the process of transitioning to a carnivore diet from various dietary backgrounds, addressing potential challenges, benefits, and strategies for success.

- **Understanding the Carnivore Diet**

The carnivore diet is an eating approach that emphasizes animal foods while excluding most plant-based foods. Followers of this diet typically consume meat, fish, eggs, and some dairy products while avoiding carbohydrates, including fruits, vegetables, grains, legumes, and processed foods. Advocates of the carnivore diet argue that it can lead to weight loss, improved metabolic health, increased energy levels, and relief from various health conditions such as autoimmune disorders and gastrointestinal issues.

- **Transitioning from a Standard Western Diet**

For individuals accustomed to a standard Western diet high in processed foods, sugars, and carbohydrates, transitioning to a carnivore diet can be a drastic change. Initially, the removal of familiar comfort foods like bread, pasta, and sugary snacks may cause withdrawal symptoms and cravings. Moreover, adjusting to a higher intake of protein and fat while reducing carbohydrate consumption can lead to digestive discomfort, such as bloating, gas, and constipation.

To ease the transition, individuals should gradually reduce carbohydrate intake while increasing their consumption of animal-based foods. Incorporating nutrient-dense sources of protein and fat, such as grass-fed beef, pastured eggs, wild-caught fish, and organ meats, can help ensure satiety and provide essential nutrients. Additionally, staying hydrated and replenishing electrolytes, especially during the initial adaptation phase, can mitigate symptoms of carbohydrate withdrawal and support overall well-being.

- **Transitioning from a Plant-Based Diet:**
Transitioning from a plant-based diet to a carnivore diet represents a significant dietary shift, both nutritionally and philosophically. Plant-based diets, characterized by their emphasis on fruits, vegetables, grains, legumes, nuts, and seeds, provide ample fiber, vitamins,

minerals, and phytonutrients while typically containing lower amounts of protein and fat. Therefore, individuals transitioning from a plant-based diet to a carnivore diet may experience challenges related to nutrient deficiencies, digestive adaptation, and psychological adjustment.

To navigate this transition effectively, individuals should focus on gradually reintroducing animal-based foods into their diet while monitoring their body's response. Incorporating small amounts of animal products, such as eggs, fish, or dairy, can help acclimate the digestive system to the higher protein and fat content present in animal foods. Additionally, prioritizing nutrient-rich animal sources, including organ meats and bone broth, can help address potential nutrient deficiencies commonly associated with plant-based diets, such as vitamin B12, iron, zinc, and omega-3 fatty acids.

- **Strategies for Success**

  Regardless of one's previous dietary pattern, transitioning to a carnivore diet requires careful planning and consideration to ensure nutritional adequacy and long-term sustainability. Some strategies for success include:

- ➤ **Gradual Transition:** Rather than abruptly eliminating all plant-based foods, gradually reduce carbohydrate intake while increasing consumption of animal-based foods to allow the body time to adapt.

➤ **Focus on Nutrient Density:** Prioritize nutrient-dense animal sources, including grass-fed meat, pastured eggs, wild-caught fish, organ meats, and bone broth, to ensure adequate intake of essential nutrients.

➤ **Stay Hydrated:** Drink plenty of water and consider incorporating electrolyte-rich beverages, such as bone broth or electrolyte supplements, to support hydration and mineral balance.

➤ **Listen to Your Body:** Pay attention to your body's signals and adjust your dietary choices accordingly. Experiment with different foods to identify what works best for your individual needs and preferences.

➢ **Seek Professional Guidance:** Consult with a healthcare provider or registered dietitian familiar with the carnivore diet to ensure that your nutritional needs are met and to address any potential concerns or challenges.

Transitioning to a carnivore diet from other dietary patterns requires careful planning, patience, and flexibility. While the process may present challenges, including physiological adaptation, nutrient adequacy, and psychological adjustment, many individuals report experiencing significant improvements in weight, metabolic health, gut function, and energy levels on a carnivore diet. By gradually transitioning, focusing on nutrient-dense animal sources, staying hydrated, listening to your body, and seeking professional guidance when needed, individuals can successfully navigate the transition to a carnivore diet and reap its potential benefits for overall health and well-being.

Kitchen Essentials for Carnivore Cooking

Cooking on a carnivore diet revolves around animal-based ingredients, requiring a different set of kitchen essentials compared to other dietary patterns. Whether you're a seasoned carnivore enthusiast or just starting on this journey, having the right tools and equipment can enhance your cooking experience and support your dietary goals. In this part, we'll explore the essential kitchen items for carnivore cooking, including appliances, utensils, and pantry staples, to help you prepare delicious and nutrient-dense meals.

1. High-Quality Cookware

Investing in high-quality cookware is essential for carnivore cooking, as it allows you to cook meat, fish, and other animal products evenly and efficiently. Key items to have in your kitchen include:

➢ **Cast Iron Skillet:** A cast iron skillet is versatile and durable, ideal for searing steaks, frying eggs, and roasting meats. It retains heat well and can withstand high temperatures, making it perfect for carnivore cooking.

➢ **Stainless Steel Pan:** Stainless steel pans are non-reactive and easy to clean, making them suitable for cooking delicate proteins like fish and poultry. Look for pans with a heavy bottom for even heat distribution.

➢ **Grill Pan or Outdoor Grill:** A grill pan or outdoor grill allows you to achieve the classic charred flavor and grill marks on meats without the need for an outdoor barbecue. It's great for cooking steaks, burgers, and sausages.

2. Sharp Knives and Cutting Boards

Sharp knives are indispensable tools in any kitchen, especially when working with meat and other animal products. Invest in high-quality knives and cutting boards to make meal preparation safe and efficient. Key items include:

➢ **Chef's Knife:** A versatile chef's knife is essential for slicing, dicing, and chopping meat, vegetables, and herbs. Choose a knife with a comfortable handle and a sharp blade that holds its edge well.

➢ **Paring Knife:** A paring knife is useful for trimming fat, peeling vegetables, and performing detailed tasks that require precision.

➢ **Cutting Boards:** Use separate cutting boards for meat and vegetables to prevent cross-contamination. Opt for cutting boards made of wood or plastic that are easy to clean and sanitize.

3. Meat Thermometer

A meat thermometer is an indispensable tool for carnivore cooking, ensuring that your meats are cooked to the desired level of doneness while maintaining their juiciness and flavor. Look for a digital meat thermometer with a probe for accurate temperature readings. This is particularly important when cooking large cuts of meat like roasts and whole chickens to avoid undercooking or overcooking.

4. Food Processor or Blender

While not strictly necessary, a food processor or blender can be helpful for preparing carnivore-friendly sauces, dips, and dressings. Use it to blend herbs, spices, and fats to create flavorful accompaniments for your meat dishes. Additionally, a food processor can be used to grind meat at home, allowing you to control the quality and texture of your ground meat.

5. Slow Cooker or Instant Pot

A slow cooker or Instant Pot can be invaluable tools for carnivore cooking, especially for busy individuals who want to enjoy tender, flavorful meats with minimal hands-on cooking time. Use it to slow-cook tough cuts of meat like beef brisket, pork shoulder, or lamb shanks until they are melt-in-your-mouth tender. The Instant Pot, in particular, offers the added convenience of pressure cooking, allowing you to prepare meals quickly without sacrificing flavor or texture.

6. Spice Grinder or Mortar and Pestle

While the carnivore diet typically emphasizes simple seasoning with salt and pepper, adding herbs and spices can enhance the flavor of your meat dishes. Invest in a spice grinder or mortar and pestle to grind whole spices fresh for maximum flavor. Experiment with herbs like rosemary, thyme, and oregano, as well as spices like garlic powder, onion powder, and paprika to add depth and complexity to your carnivore meals.

7. Pantry Staples

Stocking your pantry with essential ingredients ensures that you always have the necessary components to whip up delicious carnivore meals. Some key pantry staples for carnivore cooking include:

➢ **Salt:** Salt is a crucial seasoning in carnivore cooking, enhancing the natural flavors of meat and other animal products. Opt for high-quality sea salt or Himalayan pink salt for best results.

➢ **Animal Fats:** Animal fats like tallow, lard, and duck fat are excellent cooking fats for carnivore diets, providing flavor and moisture to your meat dishes. Render your own animal fats at home or purchase them from reputable sources.

➢ **Bone Broth:** Bone broth is a nutrient-dense beverage that can be enjoyed on its own or used as a base for soups, stews, and sauces. Make your own bone broth using leftover bones from meat or poultry, or purchase high-quality bone broth from specialty stores.

➢ **Eggs:** Eggs are a versatile and nutritious staple in the carnivore diet, providing protein, fat, and essential vitamins and minerals. Use eggs to make omelets, frittatas, or egg cups, or enjoy them boiled, poached, or scrambled.

➤ **Herbs and Spices:** While not strictly necessary, herbs and spices can add flavor and variety to your carnivore meals. Experiment with different herbs and spices to find combinations that complement your favorite meats.

8. Storage Containers

Proper storage containers are essential for storing leftovers, meal prepping, and organizing your carnivore ingredients. Invest in a variety of containers in different sizes and shapes to accommodate various portion sizes and food items. Look for containers that are microwave-safe, dishwasher-safe, and freezer-safe for maximum versatility and convenience.

Having the right kitchen essentials is essential for successful carnivore cooking. From high-quality cookware and sharp knives to essential pantry staples and storage containers, each item plays a crucial role in preparing delicious and nutritious meat-based meals. Whether you're a seasoned carnivore enthusiast or just starting on your carnivore journey, investing in these kitchen essentials will help you enjoy the benefits of the carnivore diet while unleashing your culinary creativity in the kitchen.

Tips for Dining Out and Social Situations

Following a carnivore diet can present unique challenges when dining out or navigating social situations where food is involved. Whether you're attending a restaurant gathering, a family event, or a social outing with friends, sticking to your dietary preferences while maintaining social harmony requires thoughtful planning and effective communication. In this part, we'll explore practical tips and strategies for dining out and navigating social situations on a carnivore diet, empowering you to enjoy social gatherings while staying true to your dietary goals.

1. Research Restaurants in Advance

Before dining out, research restaurants in your area that offer carnivore-friendly options or are willing to accommodate special dietary requests. Look for steakhouses, barbecue joints, and seafood restaurants that specialize in high-quality animal-based dishes. Many restaurants also provide online menus, making it easier to identify suitable options ahead of time.

2. Customize Your Order

When dining out, don't hesitate to customize your order to fit your dietary preferences. Most restaurants are willing to accommodate special requests, such as omitting sauces, dressings, or side dishes that contain non-carnivore ingredients. Additionally, you can ask for substitutions, such as extra meat or eggs, to ensure that your meal is satisfying and nutritionally balanced.

3. Focus on Whole Foods

Choose dishes that feature whole, unprocessed animal foods, such as steak, chicken, fish, and eggs. Avoid dishes that contain hidden carbohydrates or additives, such as breaded meats, processed meats, and sugary sauces. Opt for simple preparations, such as grilled, roasted, or broiled meats, to minimize unnecessary ingredients and maximize flavor.

4. Communicate with Waitstaff

Communicate your dietary preferences clearly and politely with the waitstaff to ensure that your needs are understood and accommodated. Ask questions about how dishes are prepared and request modifications or substitutions as needed. Most restaurants are willing to accommodate special dietary requests, so don't be afraid to ask for what you need.

5. Be Flexible and Creative

Be open to creative solutions and flexible adaptations when dining out on a carnivore diet. For example, you can order a steak salad without the salad components or ask for a side of bacon or sausage to complement your meal. Look for menu items that can be easily modified to fit your dietary preferences, such as customizable omelets or build-your-own burger options.

6. Plan Ahead for Social Gatherings

When attending social gatherings or events where food will be served, plan ahead to ensure that you have suitable options available. If possible, offer to bring a dish or snack that aligns with your dietary preferences, such as a platter of meat and cheese or deviled eggs. This not only ensures that you have something to eat but also allows you to share your favorite carnivore-friendly foods with others.

7. Communicate with Hosts

If you're attending a gathering hosted by friends or family, communicate your dietary preferences and any food restrictions or allergies in advance. Offer to provide suggestions or recipes for carnivore-friendly dishes that the host can include in the menu. Most hosts are accommodating and understanding when it comes to dietary preferences, so don't hesitate to communicate your needs politely and respectfully.

8. Focus on Socializing

Remember that social gatherings are about more than just food. Focus on enjoying the company of friends and loved ones rather than fixating on what you can or cannot eat. Engage in meaningful conversations, participate in activities, and focus on the social aspect of the event rather than the food.

9. Bring Snacks or Supplements

If you're unsure about the availability of suitable food options at a social gathering or event, consider bringing your own snacks or supplements to ensure that you have something to eat. Pack portable carnivore-friendly snacks, such as beef jerky, hard-boiled eggs, or cheese sticks, to keep you satisfied between meals. Additionally, consider bringing supplements like electrolyte tablets or protein powder to support your nutritional needs.

10. Practice Mindful Eating

Practice mindful eating when dining out or attending social gatherings to ensure that you're making conscious choices that align with your dietary goals. Pay attention to your hunger and satiety cues, eat slowly, and savor each bite to fully appreciate the flavors and textures of your food. By practicing mindful eating, you can enjoy your meals more fully while staying in tune with your body's needs.

11. Be Prepared for Questions

Be prepared to answer questions about your dietary preferences and explain why you choose to follow a carnivore diet. Some people may be curious or skeptical about your dietary choices, so be ready to provide information and educate others about the benefits of a carnivore lifestyle. Approach questions with patience and openness, and use the opportunity to share your knowledge and experiences with others.

12. Stay True to Your Goals

Finally, stay true to your dietary goals and priorities, even in social situations where there may be pressure to deviate from your plan. Remember why you chose to follow a carnivore diet and focus on the positive impact it has on your health and well-being. Be confident in your choices and prioritize your own needs and preferences, even if they differ from those of others.

Dining out and navigating social situations on a carnivore diet requires planning, communication, and flexibility. By researching restaurants in advance, customizing your orders, communicating with waitstaff and hosts, and staying true to your goals, you can enjoy social gatherings while sticking to your dietary preferences. Remember that food is just one aspect of social interactions, and focus on the joy of connecting with others rather than stressing over what you can or cannot eat. With these tips and strategies, you can confidently navigate any dining or social situation while following a carnivore lifestyle.

Chapter 4

Exploring Carnivore Recipes: The Basics

Essential Cooking Techniques

ooking techniques are fundamental to the culinary world, shaping the taste, texture, and overall quality of dishes. When adhering to a carnivore diet, which primarily consists of animal products, mastering essential cooking techniques becomes even more crucial to ensure the best flavor and nutritional value from meat, poultry, and fish. In this part, we will explore key cooking techniques tailored to the carnivore diet, including searing, roasting, grilling, braising, and sous vide, along with their impact on taste, texture, and health.

Searing is a cooking technique that involves quickly browning the surface of meat at high temperatures. This process creates a flavorful crust while locking in juices, resulting in tender and juicy meat. To sear meat effectively, it is essential to preheat the pan until it's hot and dry the surface of the meat thoroughly to promote browning. This technique is commonly used for steaks, chops, and other cuts of meat with a significant amount of fat, enhancing their savory flavor profile.

Roasting is another indispensable technique in carnivore cooking, particularly for larger cuts of meat or whole poultry. By cooking meat in the dry heat of an oven, roasting allows for even browning and caramelization while preserving the meat's natural juices. It is essential to season the meat generously and monitor the cooking process to achieve the desired level of doneness. Roasting is a versatile method that can be applied to various cuts of beef, pork, lamb, and poultry, resulting in succulent and flavorful dishes.

Grilling is a popular cooking technique that imparts a distinct smoky flavor to meat while creating appetizing grill marks. Whether using charcoal, gas, or electric grills, the direct heat and open flame of grilling quickly cook meat, sealing in juices and enhancing its natural flavor. It is crucial to preheat the grill and oil the grates to prevent sticking and achieve beautiful grill marks. Grilling is suitable for a wide range of meats, including steaks, burgers, sausages, and kebabs, offering endless possibilities for flavorful carnivore meals.

Braising is a cooking technique that combines dry and moist heat to tenderize tough cuts of meat while infusing them with rich flavor. By first searing the meat to develop a caramelized crust, then simmering it in liquid at a low temperature for an extended period, braising transforms inexpensive cuts into tender and flavorful dishes. Common braising liquids include broth, wine, beer, or a combination thereof, along with aromatics such as onions, garlic, and herbs. Braising is ideal for cuts like beef short ribs, pork shoulder, and lamb shanks, yielding meltingly tender results that are perfect for the carnivore diet.

Sous vide, a cooking technique that has gained popularity in recent years, involves vacuum-sealing food in a plastic pouch and cooking it in a water bath at a precisely controlled temperature. This method ensures precise temperature control, resulting in evenly cooked meat with a tender and juicy texture. Sous vide is particularly well-suited for lean cuts of meat, poultry, and fish, as it minimizes the risk of overcooking and preserves their natural moisture. While sous vide requires specialized equipment, such as a sous vide immersion circulator and vacuum sealer, it offers unmatched precision and consistency in carnivore cooking.

In addition to these primary cooking techniques, there are several other methods and practices that are essential for success in carnivore cooking. **Resting meat** after cooking allows the juices to redistribute evenly, resulting in a more tender and flavorful final product. Proper seasoning with salt and pepper enhances the natural flavors of meat, while marinades and rubs can add additional depth and complexity. Using high-quality ingredients, such as grass-fed beef, pasture-raised poultry, and wild-caught fish, ensures superior flavor and nutritional value in carnivore dishes.

Moreover, understanding the principles of food safety and hygiene is paramount when working with animal products. Proper handling, storage, and cooking of meat, poultry, and fish help prevent foodborne illnesses and ensure the safety of carnivore meals. It is essential to follow guidelines for internal cooking temperatures and to clean and sanitize cooking surfaces and utensils regularly.

Mastering essential cooking techniques is essential for success in the carnivore diet, allowing individuals to prepare flavorful, tender, and nutritious meals from a variety of animal products. Whether searing, roasting, grilling, braising, or sous vide, each technique offers unique benefits and contributes to the overall enjoyment of carnivore cuisine. By combining these techniques with high-quality ingredients and proper food safety practices, carnivore enthusiasts can create delicious and satisfying dishes that support their dietary preferences and health goals.

Stocking Your Pantry and Fridge

Stocking your pantry and fridge for a carnivore diet requires careful consideration to ensure you have a variety of high-quality animal products on hand to meet your nutritional needs and culinary preferences. In this part, we will explore essential items to include in your carnivore pantry and fridge, as well as strategies for sourcing, storing, and organizing these ingredients.

- **Pantry Staples**

➢ Meat: The cornerstone of the carnivore diet, meat should be the primary focus of your pantry. Stock up on a variety of cuts, including beef, pork, lamb, poultry, and game meats, to keep your meals diverse and flavorful. Opt for grass-fed and pasture-raised options whenever possible to maximize nutritional benefits.

➢ Fish and Seafood: Incorporating fish and seafood into your diet provides essential omega-3 fatty acids and a variety of nutrients. Keep canned or frozen options such as salmon, sardines, tuna, and shrimp in your pantry for convenient meal options.

➢ Eggs: Eggs are a versatile and nutrient-dense addition to the carnivore diet, providing high-quality protein, vitamins, and minerals. Stock up on fresh eggs from pasture-raised chickens or consider purchasing powdered or liquid egg products for extended shelf life.

➢ Bone Broth: Rich in collagen, gelatin, and amino acids, bone broth is a nourishing addition to the carnivore diet. Keep shelf-stable or frozen bone broth on hand for sipping, cooking, or making soups and stews.

➢ Animal Fats: Animal fats such as tallow, lard, and duck fat are ideal for cooking and adding flavor to carnivore dishes. Render your own fat from meat trimmings or purchase high-quality options from reputable sources.

➢ Salt: Salt is a crucial seasoning for enhancing the flavor of meat and replenishing electrolytes on a carnivore diet. Choose unrefined sea salt or pink Himalayan salt for optimal mineral content and flavor.

➢ Herbs and Spices (optional): While not strictly necessary on a carnivore diet, herbs and spices can add variety and complexity to your meals. Stock up on dried herbs and spices such as black pepper, garlic powder, and rosemary for seasoning meat and adding flavor to dishes.

- **Refrigerator Essentials**

➢ Fresh Meat: Keep a selection of fresh meat in your refrigerator for immediate consumption or meal preparation. Store meat in airtight containers or sealed bags to prevent cross-contamination and spoilage.

➢ Dairy (optional): Some individuals following a carnivore diet include dairy products such as cheese, butter, and heavy cream. Choose full-fat, pasture-raised options and consume them in moderation if tolerated.

➢ Organ Meats (optional): Organ meats are nutrient powerhouses, providing essential vitamins and minerals not found in muscle meat alone. Keep fresh or frozen organ meats such as liver, heart, and kidney in your refrigerator for occasional consumption.

➢ Eggs: Store fresh eggs in the refrigerator to maintain their freshness and quality. Check the expiration date and discard any eggs that are past their prime.

➢ Condiments (optional): While most condiments are not compatible with a strict carnivore diet, some individuals may choose to include minimal amounts of low-carb options such as mustard, hot sauce, or sugar-free ketchup. Choose brands without added sugars or artificial ingredients.

➢ Leftovers: Store leftover cooked meat in the refrigerator for quick and easy meals throughout the week. Reheat leftovers gently to preserve their moisture and flavor.

• **Sourcing and Storage Tips**

➢ Quality Over Quantity: When stocking your pantry and fridge for a carnivore diet, prioritize quality over quantity. Invest in high-quality, nutrient-dense animal products from reputable sources to ensure optimal flavor and nutrition.

➤ Local and Sustainable: Whenever possible, source meat, poultry, and eggs from local farms and producers practicing sustainable and ethical farming methods. This supports local agriculture and ensures the highest standards of animal welfare and food quality.

➤ Bulk Purchasing: Consider buying meat in bulk to take advantage of cost savings and ensure you always have plenty on hand. Many farms and butcher shops offer bulk purchasing options such as quarter, half, or whole animals.

➤ Proper Storage: Proper storage is essential for maintaining the freshness and quality of meat and other perishable items. Store fresh meat in the refrigerator or freezer according to recommended storage guidelines, and use or freeze it before the expiration date.

➢ Labeling and Organization: Keep your pantry and fridge organized by labeling items with their purchase or expiration dates and arranging them in a logical manner. This makes it easier to rotate stock and avoid food waste.

➢ Freezing: Freeze meat and other perishable items if you don't plan to use them within a few days to prevent spoilage. Use airtight containers, vacuum-sealed bags, or freezer-safe wraps to minimize exposure to air and moisture.

Stocking your pantry and fridge for a carnivore diet requires careful planning and consideration to ensure you have a variety of high-quality animal products on hand to meet your nutritional needs and culinary preferences. By including essential pantry staples such as meat, fish, eggs, and bone broth, along with optional items like dairy, organ meats, and condiments, you can create delicious and satisfying carnivore meals while supporting your health and well-being. Remember to prioritize quality, source locally and sustainably whenever possible, and practice proper storage and organization to make the most of your carnivore kitchen.

Meal Planning for Success

Meal planning is a crucial component of success on any dietary regimen, including the carnivore diet. Proper meal planning ensures that you have access to nutrient-dense foods that support your health goals while minimizing the risk of nutrient deficiencies or food boredom. In this part, we will delve into the importance of meal planning for the carnivore diet, explore strategies for effective meal planning, and provide practical tips for incorporating variety and balance into carnivore meal plans.

- **Importance of Meal Planning for the Carnivore Diet**

➢ Nutritional Adequacy: Planning meals in advance allows you to ensure that your diet is nutritionally adequate, providing all essential nutrients required for optimal health. This is particularly important on the carnivore diet, which eliminates many plant-based foods that are rich sources of vitamins, minerals, and phytonutrients.

➢ Optimal Food Selection: Meal planning enables you to make informed choices about the types of foods you include in your diet, ensuring that you prioritize nutrient-dense animal products while minimizing processed foods and empty calories. By selecting high-quality meats, fish, eggs, and organ meats, you can maximize the nutritional value of your meals.

➢ Budget and Cost Savings: Planning meals in advance allows you to shop strategically, minimizing food waste and maximizing your budget. By buying ingredients in bulk, taking advantage of sales and discounts, and utilizing leftovers effectively, you can save money while following a carnivore diet.

➢ Time Efficiency: Meal planning can help streamline your cooking and meal preparation process, saving you time and effort throughout the week. By batching cooking tasks, preparing ingredients in advance, and having a plan in place, you can minimize the time spent in the kitchen while still enjoying delicious and nutritious meals.

➤ Consistency and Compliance: Following a
carnivore diet requires dedication and
consistency to reap the benefits fully. Meal
planning helps you stay on track with your
dietary goals by providing structure and
guidance, reducing the temptation to deviate
from your plan or indulge in non-compliant
foods.

- **Strategies for Effective Meal Planning on
the Carnivore Diet**

➤ Set Clear Goals: Before embarking on meal
planning, clarify your dietary goals and
preferences. Consider factors such as your
daily caloric and macronutrient needs, food
intolerances or allergies, taste preferences, and
health objectives. This will guide your meal

planning decisions and ensure that your meals align with your individual needs.

➤ Create a Weekly Meal Plan: Start by creating a weekly meal plan that outlines your meals and snacks for each day of the week. Take into account your schedule, lifestyle, and cooking abilities when planning meals, and aim for a balance of protein, fat, and micronutrients in each meal. Incorporate a variety of meats, fish, eggs, and dairy (if tolerated) to ensure nutritional diversity.

➤ Batch Cooking and Meal Prep: Batch cooking and meal prep are key strategies for efficient meal planning on the carnivore diet. Set aside time each week to cook large batches of meat, poultry, and fish, then portion them into individual servings for easy reheating throughout the week. Prepping ingredients such as chopped vegetables, seasoned meats, and homemade condiments can also streamline meal preparation and save time.

➢ Utilize Leftovers: Leftovers are a valuable resource for carnivore meal planning, allowing you to repurpose cooked meat into new dishes or enjoy quick and easy meals on busy days. Plan meals with leftovers in mind, and consider incorporating versatile ingredients that can be used in multiple dishes, such as roast chicken or slow-cooked beef.

➢ Experiment with Recipes and Flavors: While the carnivore diet may seem restrictive at first glance, there are endless possibilities for creative and flavorful meals. Experiment with different cuts of meat, cooking methods, and seasoning combinations to keep your meals interesting and satisfying. Look for carnivore-friendly recipes online or adapt traditional recipes to fit your dietary preferences.

➢ Stay Flexible: While meal planning provides structure and guidance, it's essential to remain flexible and adaptable to changes in your schedule or preferences. Allow for some flexibility in your meal plan to accommodate unexpected events or cravings, and be open to adjusting your plan as needed.

- **Practical Tips for Carnivore Meal Planning**

➢ Keep It Simple: Focus on simplicity when planning carnivore meals, emphasizing high-quality animal products prepared with minimal ingredients. Simple meals like grilled steak, roasted chicken, or pan-seared fish can be both delicious and nutritious without requiring elaborate preparation.

➢ Plan for Snacks: Incorporate carnivore-friendly snacks into your meal plan to satisfy hunger between meals and prevent overeating. Consider portable options such as beef jerky, hard-boiled eggs, canned fish, or cheese (if tolerated) for convenient on-the-go snacks.

➢ Rotate Protein Sources: To ensure nutritional diversity and prevent monotony, rotate your protein sources regularly throughout the week. Include a variety of meats, poultry, fish, and organ meats in your meal plan to provide a broad spectrum of nutrients and flavors.

➢ Focus on Quality: Quality is paramount on the carnivore diet, so prioritize high-quality, pasture-raised, and grass-fed animal products whenever possible. Choose meats and eggs from reputable sources that prioritize animal welfare and sustainable farming practices.

➢ Listen to Your Body: Pay attention to your body's hunger and satiety cues when planning meals, and adjust your portion sizes and meal frequency accordingly. Some individuals may thrive on three larger meals per day, while others may prefer smaller, more frequent meals or intermittent fasting.

➢ Plan for Social Situations: Consider how social events and dining out may fit into your meal plan, and plan accordingly. Research carnivore-friendly options at restaurants or prepare a dish to bring to gatherings to ensure that you can stick to your dietary goals while still enjoying social occasions.

Meal planning is a cornerstone of success on the carnivore diet, providing structure, guidance, and efficiency in your dietary journey. By setting clear goals, creating a weekly meal plan, utilizing batch cooking and meal prep techniques, and staying flexible and adaptable, you can streamline your carnivore meal planning process and enjoy delicious and nutritious meals that support your health and well-being. With careful planning and consideration, you can thrive on the carnivore diet while experiencing the benefits of optimal nutrition and culinary satisfaction.

Chapter 5

Delicious and Nutritious

Carnivore Breakfasts

Bacon and Eggs

Description: A classic breakfast combination of crispy bacon strips and perfectly cooked eggs, providing a savory and satisfying start to the day.

Preparation time: 5 minutes

Cooking time: 10 minutes

Ingredients:

- 4 strips of bacon

- 4 eggs

- Salt and pepper to taste

Directions:

1. Heat a skillet over medium heat and add the bacon strips.

2. Cook the bacon until crispy, flipping occasionally, about 5-7 minutes.

3. Remove the bacon from the skillet and set it aside on a plate lined with paper towels to drain excess grease.

4. In the same skillet with the bacon drippings, crack the eggs and cook them to your desired doneness, either sunny-side-up, over easy, or scrambled.

5. Season the eggs with salt and pepper to taste.

6. Serve the bacon and eggs hot, garnished with herbs if desired.

Nutritional value: (per serving)

- Calories: 320

- Protein: 17g

- Fat: 26g

- Carbohydrates: 1g

- Fiber: 0g

Steak and Eggs

Description: A hearty breakfast featuring tender, juicy steak paired with eggs, providing a protein-packed meal to kick-start your day.

Preparation time: 10 minutes

Cooking time: 15 minutes

Ingredients:

- 1 steak (ribeye, sirloin, or your preferred cut)

- 2 eggs

- Salt and pepper to taste

- Olive oil or butter for cooking

Directions:

1. Season the steak generously with salt and pepper on both sides.

2. Heat a skillet or grill pan over medium-high heat and add a drizzle of olive oil or a pat of butter.

3. Place the steak in the hot skillet and cook to your desired level of doneness, flipping halfway through, approximately 3-5 minutes per side for medium-rare.

4. While the steak is cooking, crack the eggs into the skillet and cook them to your preference alongside the steak.

5. Once the steak is cooked to your liking, remove it from the skillet and let it rest for a few minutes before slicing.

6. Serve the sliced steak with the eggs on the side, seasoned with additional salt and pepper if desired.

Nutritional value: (per serving)

- Calories: 480

- Protein: 42g

- Fat: 34g

- Carbohydrates: 1g

- Fiber: 0g

Carnivore Breakfast Bowls

Description: A satisfying breakfast bowl packed with ground beef, eggs, and cheese, providing a hearty and protein-rich meal to fuel your day.

Preparation time: 10 minutes

Cooking time: 15 minutes

Ingredients:

- 1 lb ground beef

- 4 eggs

- 1 cup shredded cheese (cheddar, mozzarella, or your favorite)

- Salt and pepper to taste

Directions:

1. In a skillet over medium heat, brown the ground beef, breaking it apart with a spatula as it cooks, until no longer pink, approximately 5-7 minutes.

2. Drain any excess grease from the skillet, if necessary.

3. Crack the eggs into the skillet with the cooked ground beef and scramble them together until the eggs are fully cooked.

4. Season the beef and eggs mixture with salt and pepper to taste.

5. Sprinkle the shredded cheese over the top of the beef and eggs mixture and allow it to melt slightly.

6. Divide the mixture into serving bowls and serve hot.

Nutritional value: (per serving)

- Calories: 530

- Protein: 45g

- Fat: 37g

- Carbohydrates: 2g

- Fiber: 0g

Breakfast Sausage Patties

Description: Homemade breakfast sausage patties seasoned to perfection, offering a flavorful and satisfying addition to your morning meal.

Preparation time: 10 minutes

Cooking time: 10 minutes

Ingredients:

- 1 lb ground pork

- 1 teaspoon salt

- 1/2 teaspoon black pepper

- 1/2 teaspoon ground sage

- 1/4 teaspoon dried thyme

- 1/4 teaspoon crushed red pepper flakes (optional)

- 1/4 teaspoon garlic powder

- 1/4 teaspoon onion powder

Directions:

1. In a large mixing bowl, combine the ground pork with all the seasoning ingredients.

2. Mix the seasonings thoroughly into the ground pork until well incorporated.

3. Divide the seasoned pork mixture into equal portions and shape them into patties.

4. Heat a skillet or griddle over medium heat and add the sausage patties.

5. Cook the patties for 4-5 minutes on each side, or until golden brown and cooked through.

6. Once cooked, remove the sausage patties from the skillet and drain on paper towels to remove excess grease.

7. Serve the sausage patties hot alongside your favorite breakfast dishes.

Nutritional value: (per serving, based on 2 patties)

- Calories: 280

- Protein: 20g

- Fat: 22g

- Carbohydrates: 1g

- Fiber: 0g

Carnivore Breakfast Casserole

Description: A hearty and satisfying breakfast casserole featuring a carnivore-friendly combination of ground beef, eggs, and cheese, baked to perfection for a flavorful morning meal.

Preparation time: 15 minutes

Cooking time: 45 minutes

Ingredients:

- 1 lb ground beef

- 8 eggs

- 1 cup shredded cheese (cheddar, mozzarella, or your favorite)

- Salt and pepper to taste

Directions:

1. Preheat your oven to 375°F (190°C) and grease a baking dish with cooking spray or butter.

2. In a skillet over medium heat, brown the ground beef, breaking it apart with a spatula as

it cooks, until no longer pink, approximately 5-7 minutes.

3. Drain any excess grease from the skillet, if necessary.

4. In a mixing bowl, whisk together the eggs and season with salt and pepper to taste.

5. Spread the cooked ground beef evenly in the greased baking dish.

6. Pour the whisked eggs over the ground beef in the baking dish.

7. Sprinkle the shredded cheese over the top of the egg and beef mixture.

8. Bake the casserole in the preheated oven for 30-35 minutes, or until the eggs are set and the cheese is melted and bubbly.

9. Once cooked, remove the casserole from the oven and let it cool slightly before slicing and serving.

Nutritional value: (per serving)

- Calories: 410

- Protein: 32g

- Fat: 28g

- Carbohydrates: 2g

- Fiber: 0g

Pork Roll, Egg, and Cheese Rolls

Description: A delicious breakfast treat featuring savory pork roll, fluffy scrambled eggs, and melted cheese rolled up in a soft tortilla, perfect for a grab-and-go morning meal.

Preparation time: 10 minutes

Cooking time: 10 minutes

Ingredients:

- 4 large eggs
- 4 slices of pork roll
- 4 slices of cheese (American, cheddar, or your favorite)
- 4 large flour tortillas
- Salt and pepper to taste

Directions:

1. In a skillet over medium heat, cook the pork roll slices until lightly browned on both sides, about 2-3 minutes per side. Set aside.

2. In the same skillet, scramble the eggs until just set, seasoning with salt and pepper to taste.

3. Lay out the flour tortillas and place a slice of cheese in the center of each tortilla.

4. Divide the scrambled eggs evenly among the tortillas, placing them on top of the cheese.

5. Place a cooked pork roll slice on top of the eggs on each tortilla.

6. Roll up the tortillas tightly to form rolls.

7. Heat a clean skillet over medium heat and lightly toast the rolls on all sides until the cheese is melted and the tortillas are golden brown.

8. Serve the pork roll, egg, and cheese rolls hot, optionally with salsa or hot sauce for dipping.

Nutritional value: (per roll)

- Calories: 390

- Protein: 18g

- Fat: 22g

- Carbohydrates: 29g

- Fiber: 1g

Baked Eggs in Ham Cups

Description: A simple and elegant breakfast dish featuring eggs baked in individual ham cups, offering a protein-packed and low-carb morning meal.

Preparation time: 10 minutes

Cooking time: 15 minutes

Ingredients:

- 8 slices of ham

- 8 large eggs

- Salt and pepper to taste

- Chopped fresh herbs for garnish (optional)

Directions:

1. Preheat your oven to 375°F (190°C) and lightly grease a muffin tin.

2. Line each muffin cup with a slice of ham, pressing it gently into the bottom and up the sides to form a cup shape.

3. Crack an egg into each ham cup.

4. Season the eggs with salt and pepper to taste.

5. Bake in the preheated oven for 12-15 minutes, or until the egg whites are set but the yolks are still slightly runny.

6. Remove the baked eggs from the muffin tin using a spoon and transfer them to serving plates.

7. Garnish with chopped fresh herbs if desired, and serve hot.

    Nutritional value: (per serving)

- Calories: 170

- Protein: 16g

- Fat: 11g

- Carbohydrates: 1g

- Fiber: 0g

Chicken Apple Sausage and Spinach Omelet

Description: A flavorful and nutritious omelet featuring chicken apple sausage and spinach, providing a protein-rich and vitamin-packed breakfast option.

Preparation time: 10 minutes

Cooking time: 10 minutes

Ingredients:

- 3 large eggs

- 2 chicken apple sausages, sliced

- 1 cup fresh spinach leaves

- Salt and pepper to taste

- Olive oil or butter for cooking

Directions:

1. In a bowl, beat the eggs and season with salt and pepper to taste.

2. Heat a skillet over medium heat and add a drizzle of olive oil or a pat of butter.

3. Add the sliced chicken apple sausages to the skillet and cook until lightly browned, about 2-3 minutes.

4. Add the fresh spinach leaves to the skillet and cook until wilted, about 1-2 minutes.

5. Pour the beaten eggs into the skillet, swirling to evenly distribute the sausage and spinach.

6. Cook the omelet until the edges begin to set, then gently lift the edges with a spatula and tilt

the skillet to allow the uncooked egg to flow underneath.

7. Once the eggs are mostly set, fold the omelet in half and cook for another minute to ensure the eggs are fully cooked through.

8. Slide the omelet onto a plate and serve hot.

Nutritional value: (per serving)

- Calories: 320

- Protein: 25g

- Fat: 22g

- Carbohydrates: 4g

- Fiber: 1g

Carnivore Breakfast Wraps

Description: A satisfying breakfast wrap filled with scrambled eggs, crispy bacon, and melted cheese, offering a protein-packed and portable morning meal.

Preparation time: 10 minutes

Cooking time: 10 minutes

Ingredients:

- 4 large eggs

- 8 slices of bacon

- 4 slices of cheese (cheddar, Swiss, or your favorite)

- 4 large low-carb tortillas

- Salt and pepper to taste

Directions:

1. In a skillet over medium heat, cook the bacon until crispy, about 5-7 minutes. Remove from the skillet and drain on paper towels.

2. In the same skillet, scramble the eggs until just set, seasoning with salt and pepper to taste.

3. Lay out the low-carb tortillas and place a slice of cheese in the center of each tortilla.

4. Divide the scrambled eggs evenly among the tortillas, placing them on top of the cheese.

5. Place two slices of cooked bacon on top of the eggs on each tortilla.

6. Roll up the tortillas tightly to form wraps.

7. Heat a clean skillet over medium heat and lightly toast the wraps on all sides until the cheese is melted and the tortillas are golden brown.

8. Serve the breakfast wraps hot, optionally with avocado slices or salsa.

Nutritional value: (per wrap)

- Calories: 380

- Protein: 20g

- Fat: 25g

- Carbohydrates: 15g

- Fiber: 7g

Prosciutto and Mushroom Omelet

Description: An elegant and flavorful omelet featuring thinly sliced prosciutto and sautéed mushrooms, offering a gourmet twist on a classic breakfast dish.

Preparation time: 10 minutes

Cooking time: 10 minutes

Ingredients:

- 3 large eggs

- 2 slices of prosciutto, thinly sliced

- 1/2 cup sliced mushrooms

- Salt and pepper to taste

- Olive oil or butter for cooking

Directions:

1. In a bowl, beat the eggs and season with salt and pepper to taste.

2. Heat a skillet over medium heat and add a drizzle of olive oil or a pat of butter.

3. Add the sliced mushrooms to the skillet and cook until golden brown and tender, about 5 minutes.

4. Remove the mushrooms from the skillet and set aside.

5. In the same skillet, add the thinly sliced prosciutto and cook until lightly crisp, about 1-2 minutes on each side. Remove from the skillet and set aside.

6. Pour the beaten eggs into the skillet, swirling to evenly distribute.

7. Cook the omelet until the edges begin to set, then gently lift the edges with a spatula and tilt the skillet to allow the uncooked egg to flow underneath.

8. Once the eggs are mostly set, place the cooked mushrooms and prosciutto slices on one half of the omelet.

9. Fold the other half of the omelet over the filling and cook for another minute to ensure the eggs are fully cooked through.

10. Slide the omelet onto a plate and serve hot.

Nutritional value: (per serving)

- Calories: 280

- Protein: 20g

- Fat: 20g

- Carbohydrates: 2g

- Fiber: 1g

Brunch Steak with Sunny Side Up Eggs

Description: A hearty brunch option featuring tender steak served with perfectly cooked sunny side up eggs, creating a satisfying and protein-rich meal.

Preparation time: 10 minutes

Cooking time: 15 minutes

Ingredients:

- 2 steak cuts of your choice (e.g., ribeye, sirloin)

- 4 large eggs

- Salt and pepper to taste

- Olive oil or butter for cooking

Directions:

1. Season the steak cuts generously with salt and pepper on both sides.

2. Heat a skillet or grill pan over medium-high heat and add a drizzle of olive oil or a pat of butter.

3. Place the steak cuts in the hot skillet and cook to your desired level of doneness, flipping halfway through, approximately 3-5 minutes per side for medium-rare.

4. While the steak is cooking, crack the eggs into the skillet and cook them sunny side up.

5. Season the eggs with salt and pepper to taste.

6. Once the steak is cooked to your liking, remove it from the skillet and let it rest for a few minutes before serving.

7. Serve the steak with the sunny side up eggs on top, and optionally with a side of toast or hash browns.

Nutritional value: (per serving)

- Calories: 480

- Protein: 38g

- Fat: 32g

- Carbohydrates: 1g

- Fiber: 0g

Carnivore Breakfast Tacos

Description: A delicious and protein-packed breakfast option featuring scrambled eggs, tender steak, and melted cheese wrapped in low-carb tortillas, perfect for a quick and satisfying morning meal.

Preparation time: 10 minutes

Cooking time: 10 minutes

Ingredients:

- 4 large eggs

- 1 cup cooked steak, diced

- 1 cup shredded cheese (cheddar, Monterey Jack, or your favorite)

- 4 large low-carb tortillas

- Salt and pepper to taste

Directions:

1. In a skillet over medium heat, scramble the eggs until just set, seasoning with salt and pepper to taste.

2. Remove the scrambled eggs from the skillet and set aside.

3. In the same skillet, warm the diced steak until heated through.

4. Lay out the low-carb tortillas and divide the scrambled eggs, diced steak, and shredded cheese evenly among them.

5. Roll up the tortillas tightly to form tacos.

6. Optional: Heat a clean skillet over medium heat and lightly toast the tacos on all sides until the cheese is melted and the tortillas are golden brown.

7. Serve the breakfast tacos hot, optionally with salsa or avocado slices.

Nutritional value: (per taco)

- Calories: 370

- Protein: 28g

- Fat: 24g

- Carbohydrates: 7g

- Fiber: 3g

Smoked Salmon and Scrambled Eggs

Description: A luxurious breakfast option featuring creamy scrambled eggs paired with delicate smoked salmon, offering a gourmet and protein-rich morning meal.

Preparation time: 5 minutes

Cooking time: 5 minutes

Ingredients:

- 4 large eggs

- 4 oz smoked salmon

- 2 tablespoons heavy cream or milk

- Salt and pepper to taste

- Chopped fresh dill for garnish (optional)

Directions:

1. In a bowl, beat the eggs with the heavy cream or milk until well combined.

2. Season the beaten eggs with salt and pepper to taste.

3. Heat a skillet over medium heat and add a pat of butter.

4. Pour the beaten eggs into the skillet and cook, stirring gently, until just set and creamy.

5. Remove the scrambled eggs from the skillet and divide them among serving plates.

6. Top each serving of scrambled eggs with smoked salmon slices.

7. Garnish with chopped fresh dill if desired, and serve hot.

Nutritional value: (per serving)

- Calories: 320

- Protein: 24g

- Fat: 22g

- Carbohydrates: 1g

- Fiber: 0g

Chorizo and Egg Breakfast Bowls

Description: A flavorful and satisfying breakfast bowl featuring spicy chorizo sausage and scrambled eggs, providing a protein-packed and flavorful morning meal.

Preparation time: 10 minutes

Cooking time: 15 minutes

Ingredients:

- 1 lb chorizo sausage, casings removed

- 8 large eggs

- Salt and pepper to taste

- 1 cup shredded cheese (cheddar, pepper jack, or your favorite)

Directions:

1. In a skillet over medium heat, cook the chorizo sausage, breaking it apart with a spatula as it cooks, until browned and cooked through, approximately 5-7 minutes.

2. In a separate bowl, beat the eggs and season with salt and pepper to taste.

3. Pour the beaten eggs into the skillet with the cooked chorizo and scramble them until just set.

4. Once the eggs are cooked, remove the skillet from the heat and sprinkle the shredded cheese over the top of the chorizo and eggs.

5. Cover the skillet and let it sit for a minute to allow the cheese to melt.

6. Divide the chorizo and egg mixture into serving bowls and serve hot.

Nutritional value: (per serving)

- Calories: 480

- Protein: 32g

- Fat: 36g

- Carbohydrates: 3g

- Fiber: 0g

Ham and Cheese Omelet

Description: A classic breakfast favorite featuring tender ham and melted cheese folded into fluffy scrambled eggs, offering a comforting and satisfying morning meal.

Preparation time: 5 minutes

Cooking time: 5 minutes

Ingredients:

- 3 large eggs

- 2 slices of ham, diced

- 1/2 cup shredded cheese (Swiss, Gruyere, or your favorite)

- Salt and pepper to taste

- Olive oil or butter for cooking

Directions:

1. In a bowl, beat the eggs and season with salt and pepper to taste.

2. Heat a skillet over medium heat and add a drizzle of olive oil or a pat of butter.

3. Pour the beaten eggs into the skillet and cook, stirring gently, until just set and slightly runny.

4. Sprinkle the diced ham and shredded cheese over one half of the cooked eggs.

5. Fold the other half of the eggs over the filling to form a half-moon shape.

6. Cook for another minute to melt the cheese and heat the ham through.

7. Slide the omelet onto a plate and serve hot.

Nutritional value: (per serving)

- Calories: 340

- Protein: 26g

- Fat: 24g

- Carbohydrates: 2g

- Fiber: 0g

Turkey Bacon and Egg Cups

Description: A healthier twist on classic bacon and eggs, featuring turkey bacon wrapped around muffin tin cups filled with eggs, creating a protein-rich and flavorful breakfast option.

Preparation time: 10 minutes

Cooking time: 15 minutes

Ingredients:

- 6 slices of turkey bacon

- 6 large eggs

- Salt and pepper to taste

- Chopped fresh chives for garnish (optional)

Directions:

1. Preheat your oven to 375°F (190°C) and grease a muffin tin with cooking spray or butter.

2. Line each muffin cup with a slice of turkey bacon, pressing it gently into the bottom and up the sides to form a cup shape.

3. Crack an egg into each bacon-lined muffin cup.

4. Season the eggs with salt and pepper to taste.

5. Bake in the preheated oven for 12-15 minutes, or until the egg whites are set but the yolks are still slightly runny.

6. Remove the bacon and egg cups from the muffin tin using a spoon and transfer them to serving plates.

7. Garnish with chopped fresh chives if desired, and serve hot.

    Nutritional value: (per serving)

- Calories: 160

- Protein: 15g

- Fat: 10g

- Carbohydrates: 1g

- Fiber: 0g

Chicken Sausage Patties and Fried Eggs

Description: A protein-packed breakfast featuring homemade chicken sausage patties paired with perfectly fried eggs, offering a flavorful and satisfying morning meal.

Preparation time: 10 minutes

Cooking time: 15 minutes

Ingredients:

- 1 lb ground chicken

- 1 teaspoon salt

- 1/2 teaspoon black pepper

- 1/2 teaspoon dried sage

- 1/2 teaspoon dried thyme

- 1/4 teaspoon crushed red pepper flakes (optional)

- 1/4 teaspoon garlic powder

- 1/4 teaspoon onion powder

- 4 large eggs

- Olive oil or butter for cooking

Directions:

1. In a large mixing bowl, combine the ground chicken with all the seasoning ingredients.

2. Mix the seasonings thoroughly into the ground chicken until well incorporated.

3. Divide the seasoned chicken mixture into equal portions and shape them into patties.

4. Heat a skillet over medium heat and add a drizzle of olive oil or a pat of butter.

5. Cook the chicken sausage patties for 4-5 minutes on each side, or until golden brown and cooked through.

6. Once the sausage patties are cooked, remove them from the skillet and set aside.

7. In the same skillet, fry the eggs to your desired level of doneness.

8. Serve the chicken sausage patties with the fried eggs on top, and optionally with a side of toast or breakfast potatoes.

Nutritional value: (per serving)

- Calories: 320

- Protein: 28g

- Fat: 20g

- Carbohydrates: 1g

- Fiber: 0g

Corned Beef Hash with Eggs

Description: A comforting and hearty breakfast dish featuring homemade corned beef hash topped with fried or poached eggs, offering a satisfying and flavorful morning meal.

Preparation time: 15 minutes

Cooking time: 30 minutes

Ingredients:

- 2 cups cooked corned beef, diced

- 2 cups cooked potatoes, diced

- 1 onion, chopped

- 2 tablespoons butter

- Salt and pepper to taste

- 4 large eggs

Directions:

1. In a skillet over medium heat, melt the butter and add the chopped onion. Cook until translucent, about 5 minutes.

2. Add the diced corned beef and potatoes to the skillet, spreading them out evenly.

3. Season with salt and pepper to taste, and cook, stirring occasionally, until the hash is heated through and starting to crisp up, about 15-20 minutes.

4. Meanwhile, fry or poach the eggs to your desired level of doneness.

5. Once the corned beef hash is cooked, divide it among serving plates.

6. Top each serving of corned beef hash with a fried or poached egg.

7. Serve hot, optionally with a side of toast or breakfast biscuits.

Nutritional value: (per serving)

- Calories: 420

- Protein: 26g

- Fat: 28g

- Carbohydrates: 15g

- Fiber: 2g

Bacon Muffin Cups

Description: A delightful breakfast treat featuring crispy bacon wrapped around muffin tin cups filled with eggs, creating individual servings of deliciousness that are perfect for a grab-and-go morning meal.

Preparation time: 10 minutes

Cooking time: 20 minutes

Ingredients:

- 6 slices of bacon

- 6 large eggs

- Salt and pepper to taste

- Chopped fresh parsley for garnish (optional)

Directions:

1. Preheat your oven to 375°F (190°C) and grease a muffin tin with cooking spray or butter.

2. Line each muffin cup with a slice of bacon, pressing it gently into the bottom and up the sides to form a cup shape.

3. Crack an egg into each bacon-lined muffin cup.

4. Season the eggs with salt and pepper to taste.

5. Bake in the preheated oven for 15-20 minutes, or until the bacon is crispy and the egg whites are set but the yolks are still slightly runny.

6. Remove the bacon and egg cups from the muffin tin using a spoon and transfer them to serving plates.

7. Garnish with chopped fresh parsley if desired, and serve hot.

    Nutritional value: (per serving)

- Calories: 190

- Protein: 12g

- Fat: 15g

- Carbohydrates: 1g

- Fiber: 0g

Eggs Benedict with Smoked Salmon

Description: A luxurious twist on the classic Eggs Benedict, featuring perfectly poached eggs and smoked salmon atop English muffins, drizzled with hollandaise sauce, creating an elegant and flavorful breakfast dish.

Preparation time: 15 minutes

Cooking time: 15 minutes

Ingredients:

- 4 large eggs

- 4 slices of smoked salmon

- 2 English muffins, split and toasted

- Hollandaise sauce (store-bought or homemade)

- Chopped fresh chives for garnish (optional)

Directions:

1. Prepare the hollandaise sauce according to the package instructions or your preferred recipe.

2. Poach the eggs until the whites are set and the yolks are still runny.

3. Place a slice of smoked salmon on each toasted English muffin half.

4. Top each smoked salmon slice with a poached egg.

5. Drizzle hollandaise sauce over the poached eggs.

6. Garnish with chopped fresh chives if desired, and serve immediately.

Nutritional value: (per serving)

- Calories: 340

- Protein: 22g

- Fat: 18g

- Carbohydrates: 25g

- Fiber: 1g

Chapter 6

Savoring Carnivore Lunches

Ribeye Steak with Butter

Description: A juicy ribeye steak cooked to perfection and served with a flavorful butter topping.

Preparation time: 10 minutes

Cooking time: 10-15 minutes

Ingredients:

- 2 ribeye steaks

- Salt and pepper to taste

- 2 tablespoons butter

- 2 cloves garlic, minced

- 1 tablespoon fresh parsley, chopped (optional)

Directions:

1. Preheat your grill or skillet to high heat.

2. Season the ribeye steaks generously with salt and pepper on both sides.

3. Place the steaks on the grill or skillet and cook for 4-5 minutes on each side for medium-rare, or adjust the cooking time according to your desired doneness.

4. In a small saucepan, melt the butter over medium heat. Add the minced garlic and cook for 1-2 minutes until fragrant.

5. Once the steaks are done cooking, transfer them to a plate and let them rest for a few minutes.

6. Spoon the garlic butter over the steaks and sprinkle with chopped parsley if desired.

7. Serve hot and enjoy!

Nutritional value:

- Calories: 600

- Protein: 45g

- Fat: 45g

- Carbohydrates: 0g

- Fiber: 0g

Grilled Chicken Thighs

Description: Tender and flavorful grilled chicken thighs perfect for any barbecue or weeknight dinner.

Preparation time: 5 minutes

Cooking time: 20 minutes

Ingredients:

- 4 bone-in, skin-on chicken thighs

- Salt and pepper to taste

- 2 tablespoons olive oil

- 1 teaspoon paprika

- 1 teaspoon garlic powder

- 1 teaspoon onion powder

- Fresh herbs for garnish (optional)

Directions:

1. Preheat your grill to medium-high heat.

2. Pat the chicken thighs dry with paper towels and season them with salt, pepper, paprika, garlic powder, and onion powder.

3. Drizzle olive oil over the chicken thighs and rub the seasoning into the meat.

4. Place the chicken thighs on the preheated grill, skin-side down, and cook for 8-10 minutes.

5. Flip the chicken thighs and continue grilling for another 8-10 minutes, or until the internal temperature reaches 165°F (75°C).

6. Remove the chicken thighs from the grill and let them rest for a few minutes before serving.

7. Garnish with fresh herbs if desired and serve hot.

Nutritional value:

- Calories: 300

- Protein: 25g

- Fat: 20g

- Carbohydrates: 0g

- Fiber: 0g

Bacon and Eggs

Description: A classic breakfast dish featuring crispy bacon and perfectly cooked eggs.

Preparation time: 5 minutes

Cooking time: 10 minutes

Ingredients:

- 4 strips of bacon

- 4 eggs

- Salt and pepper to taste

- Chopped chives or parsley for garnish (optional)

Directions:

1. Heat a skillet over medium heat and add the bacon strips. Cook until crispy, flipping occasionally, for about 5-7 minutes.

2. Remove the bacon from the skillet and place it on a paper towel-lined plate to drain excess grease.

3. In the same skillet, crack the eggs and cook them to your desired doneness (fried, scrambled, or poached).

4. Season the eggs with salt and pepper.

5. Once the eggs are cooked, remove them from the skillet and serve alongside the crispy bacon.

6. Garnish with chopped chives or parsley if desired.

7. Serve hot with toast or your favorite breakfast sides.

Nutritional value:

- Calories: 250

- Protein: 15g

- Fat: 20g

- Carbohydrates: 1g

- Fiber: 0g

Beef Liver and Onions

Description: A hearty and nutritious dish featuring tender beef liver cooked with caramelized onions.

Preparation time: 10 minutes

Cooking time: 15 minutes

Ingredients:

- 1 lb beef liver, sliced

- Salt and pepper to taste

- 2 tablespoons butter or oil

- 2 onions, thinly sliced

- 2 cloves garlic, minced

- 1 teaspoon dried thyme (optional)

- 1 tablespoon balsamic vinegar (optional)

Directions:

1. Season the beef liver slices with salt and pepper on both sides.

2. Heat a skillet over medium heat and add the butter or oil.

3. Add the sliced onions to the skillet and cook, stirring occasionally, until caramelized, about 10-12 minutes.

4. Push the onions to the side of the skillet and add the beef liver slices. Cook for 2-3 minutes on each side, or until browned but still pink in the middle.

5. Add the minced garlic and dried thyme to the skillet and cook for another minute until fragrant.

6. If using, deglaze the skillet with balsamic vinegar, scraping up any browned bits from the bottom of the pan.

7. Serve the beef liver and onions hot, accompanied by mashed potatoes or your favorite side dishes.

Nutritional value:

- Calories: 250

- Protein: 30g

- Fat: 10g

- Carbohydrates: 10g

- Fiber: 2g

Pork Chops

Description: Juicy and flavorful pork chops seasoned and cooked to perfection.

Preparation time: 5 minutes

Cooking time: 15 minutes

Ingredients:

- 4 pork chops

- Salt and pepper to taste

- 2 tablespoons olive oil

- 2 cloves garlic, minced

- 1 teaspoon dried rosemary

- 1 teaspoon dried thyme

Directions:

1. Season the pork chops generously with salt and pepper on both sides.

2. Heat a skillet over medium-high heat and add the olive oil.

3. Add the pork chops to the skillet and cook for 5-7 minutes on each side, or until golden brown and cooked through.

4. During the last few minutes of cooking, add the minced garlic, dried rosemary, and dried thyme to the skillet, and cook until fragrant.

5. Remove the pork chops from the skillet and let them rest for a few minutes before serving.

6. Serve hot with your favorite side dishes, such as roasted vegetables or mashed potatoes.

Nutritional value:

- Calories: 300

- Protein: 25g

- Fat: 20g

- Carbohydrates: 0g

- Fiber: 0g

Lamb Chops

Description: Succulent lamb chops seasoned with aromatic herbs and spices, then grilled or pan-seared to perfection.

Preparation time: 10 minutes

Cooking time: 10-12 minutes

Ingredients:

- 4 lamb chops

- Salt and pepper to taste

- 2 tablespoons olive oil

- 2 cloves garlic, minced

- 1 teaspoon dried rosemary

- 1 teaspoon dried thyme

- 1 tablespoon fresh mint leaves, chopped (optional)

Directions:

1. Preheat your grill or skillet to medium-high heat.

2. Season the lamb chops generously with salt and pepper on both sides.

3. Drizzle olive oil over the lamb chops and rub them with minced garlic, dried rosemary, and dried thyme.

4. Place the lamb chops on the grill or skillet and cook for 5-6 minutes on each side for medium-rare, or adjust the cooking time according to your preference.

5. Remove the lamb chops from the heat and let them rest for a few minutes.

6. Garnish with fresh mint leaves if desired before serving.

7. Serve hot with your favorite side dishes, such as roasted vegetables or couscous.

Nutritional value:

- Calories: 350

- Protein: 30g

- Fat: 25g

- Carbohydrates: 0g

- Fiber: 0g

Salmon Fillet

Description: Tender and flaky salmon fillet seasoned with herbs and spices, then baked or grilled to perfection.

Preparation time: 5 minutes

Cooking time: 12-15 minutes

Ingredients:

- 4 salmon fillets

- Salt and pepper to taste

- 2 tablespoons olive oil

- 2 tablespoons lemon juice

- 2 cloves garlic, minced

- 1 teaspoon dried dill

- 1 teaspoon paprika

- Lemon wedges for serving (optional)

Directions:

1. Preheat your oven to 400°F (200°C) or grill to medium-high heat.

2. Season the salmon fillets with salt and pepper on both sides.

3. In a small bowl, whisk together olive oil, lemon juice, minced garlic, dried dill, and paprika.

4. Place the salmon fillets on a baking sheet lined with parchment paper or directly on the grill grate.

5. Brush the seasoned olive oil mixture over the salmon fillets.

6. Bake in the preheated oven or grill for 12-15 minutes, or until the salmon is cooked through and flakes easily with a fork.

7. Remove from the oven or grill and let the salmon rest for a few minutes before serving.

8. Serve hot with lemon wedges on the side if desired.

Nutritional value:

- Calories: 300

- Protein: 30g

- Fat: 20g

- Carbohydrates: 2g

- Fiber: 1g

Shrimp Scampi

Description: Succulent shrimp cooked in a garlic butter sauce with white wine and served over pasta or with crusty bread.

Preparation time: 10 minutes

Cooking time: 10 minutes

Ingredients:

- 1 lb large shrimp, peeled and deveined

- Salt and pepper to taste

- 4 tablespoons unsalted butter

- 4 cloves garlic, minced

- 1/4 cup white wine

- 2 tablespoons lemon juice

- 1 tablespoon chopped parsley

- Cooked pasta or crusty bread for serving

Directions:

1. Season the shrimp with salt and pepper.

2. In a large skillet, melt the butter over medium heat. Add the minced garlic and cook until fragrant, about 1 minute.

3. Add the shrimp to the skillet and cook until pink and opaque, about 2-3 minutes per side.

4. Deglaze the skillet with white wine and lemon juice, scraping up any browned bits from the bottom of the pan.

5. Stir in the chopped parsley and season with additional salt and pepper if needed.

6. Serve the shrimp scampi hot over cooked pasta or with crusty bread for dipping.

Nutritional value:

- Calories: 250

- Protein: 25g

- Fat: 15g

- Carbohydrates: 4g

- Fiber: 0g

Turkey Breast Slices

Description: Lean and tender turkey breast slices seasoned and cooked to perfection, perfect for sandwiches or as a main dish.

Preparation time: 5 minutes

Cooking time: 15 minutes

Ingredients:

- 4 turkey breast slices

- Salt and pepper to taste

- 2 tablespoons olive oil

- 2 teaspoons dried thyme

- 2 teaspoons dried sage

Directions:

1. Season the turkey breast slices with salt, pepper, dried thyme, and dried sage on both sides.

2. Heat a skillet over medium-high heat and add the olive oil.

3. Add the turkey breast slices to the skillet and cook for 5-7 minutes on each side, or until cooked through and golden brown.

4. Remove from the skillet and let them rest for a few minutes before serving.

5. Serve hot as a main dish or use the slices for sandwiches or wraps.

Nutritional value:

- Calories: 200

- Protein: 25g

- Fat: 10g

- Carbohydrates: 0g

- Fiber: 0g

Bison Burger Patties

Description: Juicy and flavorful bison burger patties seasoned and grilled to perfection, a lean and delicious alternative to beef.

Preparation time: 10 minutes

Cooking time: 10-12 minutes

Ingredients:

- 1 lb ground bison

- Salt and pepper to taste

- 1 tablespoon Worcestershire sauce

- 1 teaspoon garlic powder

- 1 teaspoon onion powder

- 4 burger buns

- Lettuce, tomato, onion, and other toppings of choice

Directions:

1. In a mixing bowl, combine the ground bison with salt, pepper, Worcestershire sauce, garlic powder, and onion powder. Mix until well combined.

2. Divide the bison mixture into 4 equal portions and shape each portion into a patty.

3. Preheat your grill to medium-high heat.

4. Grill the bison burger patties for 5-6 minutes on each side, or until they reach your desired level of doneness.

5. Toast the burger buns on the grill for a minute or until lightly golden.

6. Assemble the burgers by placing the grilled bison patties on the toasted buns and topping with lettuce, tomato, onion, and any other desired toppings.

7. Serve hot with your favorite side dishes, such as sweet potato fries or coleslaw.

Nutritional value:

- Calories: 300

- Protein: 25g

- Fat: 20g

- Carbohydrates: 20g

- Fiber: 2g

Tuna Steaks

Description: Thick, meaty tuna steaks seasoned and seared to perfection, resulting in a tender and flavorful dish.

Preparation time: 10 minutes

Cooking time: 6-8 minutes

Ingredients:

- 4 tuna steaks

- Salt and pepper to taste

- 2 tablespoons olive oil

- 2 cloves garlic, minced

- 1 tablespoon soy sauce or tamari

- 1 tablespoon lemon juice

- 1 teaspoon sesame seeds (optional)

- Fresh herbs for garnish (optional)

Directions:

1. Pat the tuna steaks dry with paper towels and season them with salt and pepper on both sides.

2. In a small bowl, whisk together olive oil, minced garlic, soy sauce or tamari, and lemon juice.

3. Heat a skillet over high heat and add the seasoned tuna steaks.

4. Sear the tuna steaks for 2-3 minutes on each side for rare to medium-rare, or adjust the cooking time according to your preference.

5. Brush the tuna steaks with the soy sauce mixture while cooking.

6. Once done, remove the tuna steaks from the skillet and let them rest for a few minutes.

7. Garnish with sesame seeds and fresh herbs if desired before serving.

8. Serve hot with steamed vegetables or a side salad.

Nutritional value:

- Calories: 250

- Protein: 30g

- Fat: 15g

- Carbohydrates: 1g

- Fiber: 0g

Sardines in Olive Oil

Description: Tender sardines preserved in flavorful olive oil, perfect for serving as an appetizer or adding to salads and pasta dishes.

Preparation time: 5 minutes

Ingredients:

- 2 cans sardines in olive oil

- Lemon wedges for serving (optional)

- Crusty bread for serving (optional)

Directions:

1. Open the cans of sardines and drain off any excess olive oil.

2. Arrange the sardines on a serving platter.

3. Serve with lemon wedges and crusty bread on the side if desired.

4. Enjoy as a simple appetizer or use the sardines to add flavor to salads, pasta dishes, or sandwiches.

Nutritional value:

- Calories: 200

- Protein: 20g

- Fat: 15g

- Carbohydrates: 0g

- Fiber: 0g

Venison Stew

Description: A hearty and comforting stew made with tender venison meat, vegetables, and aromatic herbs and spices.

Preparation time: 15 minutes

Cooking time: 2-3 hours

Ingredients:

- 1 lb venison stew meat, cubed

- Salt and pepper to taste

- 2 tablespoons olive oil

- 2 onions, chopped

- 3 carrots, chopped

- 3 celery stalks, chopped

- 4 cloves garlic, minced

- 1 tablespoon tomato paste

- 4 cups beef or vegetable broth

- 2 bay leaves

- 1 teaspoon dried thyme

- 1 teaspoon dried rosemary

- 1 cup red wine (optional)

- Chopped parsley for garnish (optional)

Directions:

1. Season the cubed venison meat with salt and pepper.

2. Heat olive oil in a large pot or Dutch oven over medium-high heat.

3. Add the venison meat to the pot and cook until browned on all sides, about 5-7 minutes.

4. Remove the venison meat from the pot and set aside.

5. In the same pot, add chopped onions, carrots, and celery. Cook until softened, about 5 minutes.

6. Add minced garlic and tomato paste to the pot. Cook for another minute until fragrant.

7. Return the browned venison meat to the pot.

8. Pour in beef or vegetable broth and add bay leaves, dried thyme, and dried rosemary.

9. If using, pour in red wine to deglaze the pot.

10. Bring the stew to a boil, then reduce the heat to low, cover, and simmer for 2-3 hours, stirring occasionally, until the venison is tender.

11. Once done, remove the bay leaves and adjust the seasoning if needed.

12. Serve hot, garnished with chopped parsley if desired, alongside crusty bread or mashed potatoes.

Nutritional value:

- Calories: 300

- Protein: 25g

- Fat: 15g

- Carbohydrates: 10g

- Fiber: 2g

Duck Breast

Description: Succulent duck breast cooked to perfection, resulting in tender and flavorful slices perfect for serving as a main dish.

Preparation time: 10 minutes

Cooking time: 15 minutes

Ingredients:

- 2 duck breasts
- Salt and pepper to taste
- 1 tablespoon olive oil
- 2 cloves garlic, minced
- 1 teaspoon dried thyme
- 1 teaspoon dried rosemary
- 2 tablespoons honey or maple syrup (optional)

Directions:

1. Score the skin of the duck breasts with a sharp knife, being careful not to cut into the meat.

2. Season the duck breasts generously with salt and pepper on both sides.

3. Heat a skillet over medium-high heat and add olive oil.

4. Place the duck breasts in the skillet, skin-side down, and cook for 6-8 minutes until the skin is golden brown and crispy.

5. Flip the duck breasts and cook for another 4-5 minutes on the other side, or until the internal temperature reaches 135°F (57°C) for medium-rare or 145°F (63°C) for medium.

6. During the last minute of cooking, add minced garlic, dried thyme, and dried rosemary to the skillet. If using, drizzle honey or maple syrup over the duck breasts.

7. Remove the duck breasts from the skillet and let them rest for a few minutes before slicing.

8. Slice the duck breasts thinly and serve hot with your favorite side dishes, such as roasted vegetables or mashed potatoes.

Nutritional value:

- Calories: 400

- Protein: 25g

- Fat: 30g

- Carbohydrates: 5g

- Fiber: 0g

Bone Broth with Beef Marrow

Description: A nourishing and comforting broth made from simmering beef bones with aromatic vegetables and herbs, enriched with flavorful beef marrow.

Preparation time: 10 minutes

Cooking time: 12-24 hours

Ingredients:

- 4 lbs beef bones (such as marrow bones or knuckle bones)

- 2 onions, quartered

- 3 carrots, chopped

- 3 celery stalks, chopped

- 4 cloves garlic, smashed

- 2 bay leaves

- 1 tablespoon apple cider vinegar (optional)

- Water

- Salt and pepper to taste

- Chopped parsley for garnish (optional)

Directions:

1. Preheat your oven to 400°F (200°C).

2. Place the beef bones on a baking sheet and roast them in the preheated oven for 30-40 minutes, or until browned.

3. Transfer the roasted bones to a large stockpot or slow cooker.

4. Add quartered onions, chopped carrots, chopped celery, smashed garlic cloves, bay leaves, and apple cider vinegar (if using) to the pot.

5. Fill the pot with enough water to cover the bones and vegetables by 2 inches.

6. Bring the water to a boil, then reduce the heat to low and let the broth simmer, uncovered, for 12-24 hours. Skim off any foam or impurities that rise to the surface.

7. Once the broth has simmered for the desired time, strain it through a fine-mesh sieve or cheesecloth into a clean container.

8. If desired, scoop out the beef marrow from the bones and add it to the strained broth.

9. Season the broth with salt and pepper to taste.

10. Serve hot as a nourishing drink or use it as a base for soups, stews, or sauces.

11. Garnish with chopped parsley if desired.

Nutritional value:

- Calories: 50

- Protein: 5g

- Fat: 3g

- Carbohydrates: 2g

- Fiber: 0g

Ground Beef Stir-Fry with Butter

Description: A quick and flavorful stir-fry made with ground beef, vegetables, and a rich buttery sauce.

Preparation time: 10 minutes

Cooking time: 15 minutes

Ingredients:

- 1 lb ground beef

- Salt and pepper to taste

- 2 tablespoons butter

- 1 onion, thinly sliced

- 2 bell peppers, thinly sliced

- 2 cloves garlic, minced

- 1 tablespoon soy sauce

- 1 tablespoon Worcestershire sauce

- 1 teaspoon paprika

- Cooked rice or noodles for serving

Directions:

1. Heat a large skillet or wok over medium-high heat.

2. Add the ground beef to the skillet and cook, breaking it up with a spoon, until browned and cooked through, about 5-7 minutes.

3. Season the beef with salt and pepper to taste and transfer it to a plate.

4. In the same skillet, melt the butter over medium heat.

5. Add the sliced onion and bell peppers to the skillet and cook until softened, about 3-4 minutes.

6. Add the minced garlic to the skillet and cook for another minute until fragrant.

7. Return the cooked ground beef to the skillet and stir to combine with the vegetables.

8. Stir in soy sauce, Worcestershire sauce, and paprika, and cook for another 2-3 minutes to allow the flavors to meld.

9. Serve the ground beef stir-fry hot over cooked rice or noodles.

Nutritional value:

- Calories: 400

- Protein: 25g

- Fat: 30g

- Carbohydrates: 10g

- Fiber: 2g

Beef Kebabs

Description: Tender chunks of beef marinated in flavorful spices and grilled to perfection on skewers.

Preparation time: 20 minutes (plus marinating time)

Cooking time: 10-12 minutes

Ingredients:

- 1 lb beef sirloin or top round, cut into 1-inch cubes

- Salt and pepper to taste

- 2 tablespoons olive oil

- 2 cloves garlic, minced

- 1 teaspoon paprika

- 1 teaspoon cumin

- 1 teaspoon coriander

- 1/2 teaspoon cinnamon

- Wooden or metal skewers

Directions:

1. In a mixing bowl, combine olive oil, minced garlic, paprika, cumin, coriander, cinnamon, salt, and pepper.

2. Add the beef cubes to the marinade and toss to coat. Cover and refrigerate for at least 1 hour, or overnight for best results.

3. Preheat your grill to medium-high heat.

4. Thread the marinated beef cubes onto skewers, leaving a little space between each piece.

5. Grill the beef kebabs for 4-5 minutes on each side, or until cooked to your desired level of doneness.

6. Remove from the grill and let them rest for a few minutes before serving.

7. Serve hot with your favorite side dishes, such as grilled vegetables and rice pilaf.

Nutritional value:

- Calories: 300

- Protein: 25g

- Fat: 20g

- Carbohydrates: 2g

- Fiber: 0g

Chicken Liver Pâté

Description: A rich and creamy spread made with sautéed chicken livers, onions, and herbs, perfect for serving on crackers or crusty bread.

Preparation time: 10 minutes

Cooking time: 10 minutes

Ingredients:

- 1 lb chicken livers, trimmed

- Salt and pepper to taste

- 4 tablespoons butter

- 1 onion, finely chopped

- 2 cloves garlic, minced

- 1/4 cup brandy or cognac

- 1 teaspoon dried thyme

- 1/2 teaspoon ground allspice

- 1/4 teaspoon ground nutmeg

- 1/4 cup heavy cream

- Chopped parsley for garnish (optional)

Directions:

1. Season the chicken livers with salt and pepper.

2. In a large skillet, melt 2 tablespoons of butter over medium heat.

3. Add the chopped onion to the skillet and cook until softened, about 3-4 minutes.

4. Add the minced garlic to the skillet and cook for another minute until fragrant.

5. Increase the heat to medium-high and add the chicken livers to the skillet. Cook for 3-4 minutes on each side, or until browned on the outside but still pink in the center.

6. Remove the skillet from the heat and carefully pour in brandy or cognac. Return the skillet to the heat and cook for another minute, allowing the alcohol to evaporate.

7. Transfer the cooked chicken livers and onions to a food processor. Add dried thyme, ground allspice, ground nutmeg, and remaining butter to the food processor.

8. Pulse until smooth and creamy, adding heavy cream gradually until the desired consistency is reached.

9. Taste and adjust seasoning if needed.

10. Transfer the pâté to serving dishes and garnish with chopped parsley if desired.

11. Serve chilled or at room temperature with crackers or crusty bread.

Nutritional value:

- Calories: 200

- Protein: 15g

- Fat: 15g

- Carbohydrates: 5g

- Fiber: 1g

Smoked Mackerel

Description: Tender and flavorful mackerel fillets smoked to perfection, perfect for serving as a standalone dish or incorporating into salads, pasta, or sandwiches.

Preparation time: 5 minutes

Ingredients:

- 2 smoked mackerel fillets

- Lemon wedges for serving (optional)

- Crusty bread or crackers for serving (optional)

Directions:

1. Remove the skin from the smoked mackerel fillets if desired.

2. Arrange the mackerel fillets on a serving platter.

3. Serve with lemon wedges and crusty bread or crackers on the side if desired.

4. Enjoy the smoked mackerel as a standalone dish or use it to add flavor to salads, pasta, or sandwiches.

Nutritional value:

- Calories: 250

- Protein: 20g

- Fat: 15g

- Carbohydrates: 0g

- Fiber: 0g

Pork Belly Slices

Description: Succulent slices of pork belly seasoned and cooked to perfection, resulting in crispy skin and tender meat.

Preparation time: 10 minutes

Cooking time: 2-3 hours

Ingredients:

- 1 lb pork belly slices

- Salt and pepper to taste

- 2 tablespoons olive oil

- 2 cloves garlic, minced

- 1 tablespoon soy sauce

- 1 tablespoon honey or maple syrup (optional)

Directions:

1. Preheat your oven to 300°F (150°C).

2. Season the pork belly slices with salt and pepper on both sides.

3. Heat olive oil in a large ovenproof skillet over medium-high heat.

4. Add the pork belly slices to the skillet, skin-side down, and cook for 5-7 minutes until the skin is golden brown and crispy.

5. Flip the pork belly slices and cook for another 2-3 minutes on the other side.

6. Add minced garlic, soy sauce, and honey or maple syrup (if using) to the skillet.

7. Transfer the skillet to the preheated oven and roast for 2-3 hours, or until the pork belly is tender and cooked through.

8. Remove from the oven and let the pork belly slices rest for a few minutes before serving.

9. Slice the pork belly and serve hot with your favorite side dishes, such as steamed rice and stir-fried vegetables.

Nutritional value:

- Calories: 400

- Protein: 20g

- Fat: 35g

- Carbohydrates: 2g

- Fiber: 0g

Chapter 7

Delicious Dinners

Perfectly Seared Ribeye Steak with Grass-Fed Butter

Description: Indulge in the succulent flavor of ribeye steak perfectly seared to a juicy medium-rare, finished with a dollop of grass-fed butter for a rich, savory taste.

Preparation time: 10 minutes

Cooking time: 10 minutes

Ingredients:

- 2 ribeye steaks, 1-inch thick

- Salt and freshly ground black pepper

- 2 tablespoons grass-fed butter

Directions:

1. Preheat a cast-iron skillet over high heat until smoking hot.

2. Season the ribeye steaks generously with salt and freshly ground black pepper on both sides.

3. Place the steaks in the skillet and cook for 3-4 minutes on each side for medium-rare, adjusting the time according to your desired level of doneness.

4. Remove the steaks from the skillet and let them rest for 5 minutes.

5. Top each steak with a tablespoon of grass-fed butter and let it melt over the hot meat.

6. Serve immediately and enjoy the perfectly seared ribeye steak with grass-fed butter.

Nutritional value: (per serving)

- Calories: 450

- Protein: 35g

- Fat: 35g

- Carbohydrates: 0g

Easy Air Fryer Carnivore Meatballs

Description: These carnivore meatballs are easy to make and perfect for a quick, protein-packed meal. Cooked in the air fryer, they come out juicy and flavorful every time.

Preparation time: 15 minutes

Cooking time: 15 minutes

Ingredients:

- 1 pound ground beef

- Salt and pepper to taste

Directions:

1. Preheat your air fryer to 375°F (190°C).

2. In a mixing bowl, combine the ground beef with salt and pepper.

3. Form the seasoned ground beef into meatballs, about 1 inch in diameter.

4. Place the meatballs in the air fryer basket, making sure they are not touching each other.

5. Cook for 12-15 minutes, or until the meatballs are browned and cooked through.

6. Remove from the air fryer and let them cool slightly before serving.

Nutritional value: (per serving)

- Calories: 250

- Protein: 25g

- Fat: 16g

- Carbohydrates: 0g

Loaded Carnivore Nachos

Description: Enjoy the ultimate carnivore snack with these loaded nachos, featuring crispy pork rinds topped with seasoned ground beef, melted cheese, and your favorite carnivore-friendly toppings.

Preparation time: 10 minutes

Cooking time: 10 minutes

Ingredients:

- 2 cups pork rinds

- 1 pound ground beef

- Salt and pepper to taste

- 1 cup shredded cheddar cheese

- Carnivore-friendly toppings (e.g., diced avocado, sliced jalapenos, chopped bacon)

Directions:

1. Preheat your oven to 350°F (175°C).

2. Spread the pork rinds in a single layer on a baking sheet.

3. In a skillet, cook the ground beef over medium heat until browned, breaking it apart with a spoon as it cooks. Season with salt and pepper to taste.

4. Spoon the cooked ground beef evenly over the pork rinds.

5. Sprinkle the shredded cheddar cheese over the ground beef.

6. Place the baking sheet in the oven and bake for 5-7 minutes, or until the cheese is melted and bubbly.

7. Remove from the oven and top with your favorite carnivore-friendly toppings.

8. Serve immediately and enjoy the loaded carnivore nachos.

Nutritional value: (per serving)

- Calories: 400

- Protein: 35g

- Fat: 28g

- Carbohydrates: 0g

Carnitas Tacos with Cilantro Lime Crema

Description: These carnitas tacos are bursting with flavor, featuring tender, slow-cooked pork, topped with a zesty cilantro lime crema, all wrapped in warm, grain-free tortillas.

Preparation time: 20 minutes

Cooking time: 4 hours

Ingredients:

For the carnitas:

- 2 pounds pork shoulder, cut into chunks

- 1 teaspoon salt

- 1 teaspoon pepper

- 1 teaspoon ground cumin

- 1 teaspoon dried oregano

- 4 cloves garlic, minced

- 1 onion, diced

- 1 orange, juiced

- 1 lime, juiced

- 1/4 cup water

- Grain-free tortillas, for serving

For the cilantro lime crema:

- 1/2 cup sour cream

- 2 tablespoons chopped fresh cilantro

- 1 tablespoon lime juice

- Salt to taste

Directions:

1. In a slow cooker, combine the pork shoulder chunks with salt, pepper, cumin, oregano, garlic, onion, orange juice, lime juice, and water.

2. Cover and cook on low for 8 hours or on high for 4 hours, until the pork is tender and easily shreds with a fork.

3. Once the pork is cooked, remove it from the slow cooker and shred it using two forks.

4. To make the cilantro lime crema, combine the sour cream, chopped cilantro, lime juice, and salt in a bowl. Mix well.

5. To assemble the tacos, warm the grain-free tortillas in a skillet or microwave.

6. Fill each tortilla with a generous portion of the shredded carnitas.

7. Drizzle the cilantro lime crema over the carnitas.

8. Serve immediately and enjoy the carnitas tacos with cilantro lime crema.

   Nutritional value: (per serving, without tortillas)

- Calories: 300

- Protein: 25g

- Fat: 20g

- Carbohydrates: 5g

Herb-Crusted Salmon

Description: Indulge in the rich flavor of salmon, coated with a savory herb crust and baked to perfection. This dish is both elegant and easy to prepare, making it perfect for a weeknight dinner or a special occasion.

Preparation time: 10 minutes

Cooking time: 15 minutes

Ingredients:

- 4 salmon fillets

- Salt and pepper to taste

- 2 tablespoons olive oil

- 1/4 cup bread crumbs (or almond flour for a keto version)

- 2 tablespoons chopped fresh parsley

- 1 tablespoon chopped fresh dill

- 1 tablespoon chopped fresh chives

- 2 cloves garlic, minced

- Lemon wedges, for serving

Directions:

1. Preheat your oven to 400°F (200°C). Line a baking sheet with parchment paper.

2. Season the salmon fillets with salt and pepper, then place them on the prepared baking sheet.

3. In a small bowl, mix together the olive oil, bread crumbs (or almond flour), chopped herbs, and minced garlic to form the herb crust.

4. Press the herb crust mixture onto the top of each salmon fillet, coating evenly.

5. Bake in the preheated oven for 12-15 minutes, or until the salmon is cooked through and flakes easily with a fork.

6. Serve hot, garnished with lemon wedges.

Nutritional value: (per serving)

- Calories: 300

- Protein: 25g

- Fat: 20g

- Carbohydrates: 5g

Creamy Tuscan Chicken

Description: This creamy Tuscan chicken dish is bursting with flavor, featuring tender chicken breasts smothered in a creamy sauce with sun-dried tomatoes, spinach, and garlic. It's a comforting and satisfying meal that's perfect for any occasion.

Preparation time: 10 minutes

Cooking time: 20 minutes

Ingredients:

- 4 boneless, skinless chicken breasts

- Salt and pepper to taste

- 2 tablespoons olive oil

- 4 cloves garlic, minced

- 1/2 cup sun-dried tomatoes, chopped

- 2 cups fresh spinach leaves

- 1 cup heavy cream

- 1/2 cup grated Parmesan cheese

- 1 teaspoon dried Italian seasoning

- Fresh basil leaves, for garnish (optional)

Directions:

1. Season the chicken breasts with salt and pepper on both sides.

2. In a large skillet, heat the olive oil over medium heat. Add the chicken breasts and cook for 6-7 minutes per side, or until golden brown and cooked through. Remove from the skillet and set aside.

3. In the same skillet, add the minced garlic and chopped sun-dried tomatoes. Cook for 1-2 minutes, until fragrant.

4. Add the fresh spinach leaves to the skillet and cook until wilted.

5. Stir in the heavy cream, grated Parmesan cheese, and dried Italian seasoning. Cook for

2-3 minutes, until the sauce has thickened slightly.

6. Return the cooked chicken breasts to the skillet, spooning the creamy sauce over the top.

7. Garnish with fresh basil leaves, if desired.

8. Serve hot, accompanied by your favorite side dishes.

Nutritional value: (per serving)

- Calories: 400

- Protein: 30g

- Fat: 25g

- Carbohydrates: 10g

One-Pan Keto Lemon Garlic Shrimp

Description: This one-pan keto lemon garlic shrimp dish is quick, easy, and bursting with bright flavors. Perfectly cooked shrimp, infused with zesty lemon and garlic, make for a delicious low-carb meal that's ready in minutes.

Preparation time: 10 minutes

Cooking time: 10 minutes

Ingredients:

- 1 pound large shrimp, peeled and deveined

- Salt and pepper to taste

- 2 tablespoons olive oil

- 4 cloves garlic, minced

- Zest of 1 lemon

- Juice of 1 lemon

- 2 tablespoons chopped fresh parsley

- Lemon wedges, for serving

Directions:

1. Season the shrimp with salt and pepper.

2. Heat the olive oil in a large skillet over medium-high heat. Add the minced garlic and cook for 1 minute, until fragrant.

3. Add the shrimp to the skillet in a single layer. Cook for 2-3 minutes per side, until pink and opaque.

4. Stir in the lemon zest, lemon juice, and chopped parsley, tossing to coat the shrimp evenly.

5. Remove from heat and serve hot, garnished with lemon wedges.

Nutritional value: (per serving)

- Calories: 200

- Protein: 25g

- Fat: 10g

- Carbohydrates: 2g

Ground Beef Casserole with Cauliflower Rice

Description: This ground beef casserole with cauliflower rice is a hearty and comforting low-carb dish that's perfect for meal prep or a family dinner. Packed with flavor and nutritious ingredients, it's sure to become a favorite in your rotation.

Preparation time: 15 minutes

Cooking time: 30 minutes

Ingredients:

- 1 pound ground beef

- 1 onion, diced

- 2 cloves garlic, minced

- 1 bell pepper, diced

- 1 teaspoon dried oregano

- 1 teaspoon dried basil

- Salt and pepper to taste

- 1 head cauliflower, riced

- 1 cup shredded cheddar cheese

- Chopped fresh parsley, for garnish (optional)

Directions:

1. Preheat your oven to 375°F (190°C).

2. In a large skillet, cook the ground beef over medium heat until browned. Drain any excess grease.

3. Add the diced onion, minced garlic, and diced bell pepper to the skillet. Cook for 3-4 minutes, until softened.

4. Season the mixture with dried oregano, dried basil, salt, and pepper.

5. Stir in the riced cauliflower and cook for an additional 5 minutes, until heated through.

6. Transfer the mixture to a greased baking dish and sprinkle the shredded cheddar cheese evenly over the top.

7. Bake in the preheated oven for 20 minutes, or until the cheese is melted and bubbly.

8. Remove from the oven and let cool slightly before serving.

9. Garnish with chopped fresh parsley, if desired.

Nutritional value: (per serving)

- Calories: 300

- Protein: 25g

- Fat: 20g

- Carbohydrates: 5g

Keto Jalapeño Popper Stuffed Chicken

Description: These keto jalapeño popper stuffed chicken breasts are a delicious twist on a classic appetizer, featuring tender chicken breasts stuffed with creamy cheese and spicy jalapeños. It's a flavorful and satisfying dish that's perfect for a low-carb dinner.

Preparation time: 15 minutes

Cooking time: 25 minutes

Ingredients:

- 4 boneless, skinless chicken breasts

- Salt and pepper to taste

- 4 ounces cream cheese, softened

- 1/2 cup shredded cheddar cheese

- 2 jalapeños, seeded and diced

- 1/4 cup almond flour

- 1 teaspoon smoked paprika

- 1 teaspoon garlic powder

- 1 teaspoon onion powder

- 1 tablespoon olive oil

Directions:

1. Preheat your oven to 375°F (190°C).

2. Using a sharp knife, cut a pocket into each chicken breast, being careful not to cut all the way through.

3. Season the chicken breasts with salt and pepper on both sides.

4. In a mixing bowl, combine the softened cream cheese, shredded cheddar cheese, and diced jalapeños.

5. Stuff each chicken breast with the cream cheese mixture, then secure the openings with toothpicks.

6. In a shallow dish, combine the almond flour, smoked paprika, garlic powder, and onion powder.

7. Dredge each stuffed chicken breast in the almond flour mixture, coating evenly.

8. Heat the olive oil in an oven-safe skillet over medium-high heat. Add the stuffed chicken breasts and cook for 3-4 minutes per side, until golden brown.

9. Transfer the skillet to the preheated oven and bake for 15-20 minutes, or until the chicken is cooked through and the cheese is melted and bubbly.

10. Remove from the oven and let cool slightly before serving.

Nutritional value: (per serving)

- Calories: 350

- Protein: 30g

- Fat: 20g

- Carbohydrates: 5g

Instant Pot Pulled Pork

Description: This Instant Pot pulled pork recipe yields tender, juicy pulled pork with minimal effort. Perfectly seasoned and cooked to perfection, it's ideal for sandwiches, tacos, salads, or any dish that craves the savory flavor of pulled pork.

Preparation time: 10 minutes

Cooking time: 90 minutes (plus time for pressure release)

Ingredients:

- 3-4 pounds pork shoulder or pork butt, trimmed of excess fat and cut into chunks

- Salt and pepper to taste

- 1 tablespoon smoked paprika

- 1 tablespoon garlic powder

- 1 tablespoon onion powder

- 1 cup chicken broth or water

- 1/2 cup apple cider vinegar

- 1/4 cup low-carb barbecue sauce (optional)

Directions:

1. Season the pork chunks generously with salt, pepper, smoked paprika, garlic powder, and onion powder.

2. Pour the chicken broth (or water) and apple cider vinegar into the Instant Pot.

3. Place the seasoned pork chunks in the Instant Pot.

4. Close the lid and set the Instant Pot to cook on high pressure for 60 minutes.

5. Once the cooking time is complete, allow the pressure to release naturally for about 15-20 minutes, then carefully release any remaining pressure manually.

6. Remove the pork from the Instant Pot and shred it using two forks.

7. If desired, mix in the low-carb barbecue sauce for added flavor.

8. Serve the pulled pork hot, with your favorite side dishes or as a filling for sandwiches, tacos, or salads.

Nutritional value: (per serving, without barbecue sauce)

- Calories: 250

- Protein: 25g

- Fat: 15g

- Carbohydrates: 0g

Keto Chili

Description: This keto-friendly chili is hearty, flavorful, and perfect for cozy nights in. Packed with ground beef, tomatoes, and spices, it's a comforting meal that's low in carbs but high in taste.

Preparation time: 15 minutes

Cooking time: 30 minutes

Ingredients:

- 1 pound ground beef

- 1 onion, diced

- 2 cloves garlic, minced

- 1 bell pepper, diced

- 1 can (14 ounces) diced tomatoes

- 1 can (8 ounces) tomato sauce

- 2 tablespoons chili powder

- 1 teaspoon ground cumin

- 1 teaspoon paprika

- Salt and pepper to taste

- Chopped fresh cilantro, for garnish (optional)

- Sour cream, for serving (optional)

- Shredded cheddar cheese, for serving (optional)

- Sliced green onions, for serving (optional)

Directions:

1. In a large pot or Dutch oven, cook the ground beef over medium heat until browned.

2. Add the diced onion, minced garlic, and diced bell pepper to the pot. Cook for 3-4 minutes, until softened.

3. Stir in the diced tomatoes, tomato sauce, chili powder, ground cumin, paprika, salt, and pepper.

4. Bring the mixture to a simmer and cook for 20-25 minutes, stirring occasionally, until the flavors are well combined and the chili has thickened.

5. Taste and adjust the seasoning as needed.

6. Serve hot, garnished with chopped fresh cilantro, sour cream, shredded cheddar cheese, and sliced green onions, if desired.

Nutritional value: (per serving)

- Calories: 300

- Protein: 25g

- Fat: 20g

- Carbohydrates: 5g (net carbs)

Beef and Broccoli Stir-Fry

Description: This beef and broccoli stir-fry is a quick and flavorful dish that's perfect for busy weeknights. Tender slices of beef, crisp broccoli florets, and a savory sauce come together in this easy-to-make recipe.

Preparation time: 15 minutes

Cooking time: 15 minutes

Ingredients:

- 1 pound flank steak, thinly sliced against the grain

- 2 tablespoons soy sauce or tamari (for gluten-free)

- 1 tablespoon sesame oil

- 2 cloves garlic, minced

- 1 teaspoon grated ginger

- 1 tablespoon olive oil or avocado oil

- 2 cups broccoli florets

- Salt and pepper to taste

- Sesame seeds, for garnish (optional)

- Sliced green onions, for garnish (optional)

- Cauliflower rice or steamed rice, for serving

Directions:

1. In a bowl, marinate the thinly sliced flank steak with soy sauce (or tamari), sesame oil, minced garlic, and grated ginger. Set aside for 10-15 minutes.

2. Heat the olive oil (or avocado oil) in a large skillet or wok over medium-high heat.

3. Add the marinated beef slices to the skillet in a single layer. Cook for 1-2 minutes without stirring, allowing the beef to sear and develop a golden brown crust.

4. Stir in the broccoli florets and cook for an additional 3-4 minutes, until the broccoli is tender-crisp and the beef is cooked to your desired level of doneness.

5. Season with salt and pepper to taste.

6. Remove from heat and garnish with sesame seeds and sliced green onions, if desired.

7. Serve hot, accompanied by cauliflower rice or steamed rice.

Nutritional value: (per serving)

- Calories: 250

- Protein: 25g

- Fat: 15g

- Carbohydrates: 5g

Keto Chicken Fried Steak

Description: This keto chicken fried steak is a low-carb version of a classic Southern dish, featuring tenderized cube steak coated in a crispy, seasoned coating. It's served with a creamy country gravy for a comforting and satisfying meal.

Preparation time: 15 minutes

Cooking time: 20 minutes

Ingredients:

For the chicken fried steak:

- 4 cube steaks

- Salt and pepper to taste

- 1/2 cup almond flour

- 1/4 cup grated Parmesan cheese

- 1 teaspoon garlic powder

- 1 teaspoon onion powder

- 1/2 teaspoon paprika

- 2 eggs, beaten

- 2 tablespoons olive oil or avocado oil

  For the country gravy:

- 2 tablespoons butter

- 2 tablespoons almond flour

- 1 cup beef broth

- Salt and pepper to taste

  Directions:

1. Season the cube steaks with salt and pepper on both sides.

2. In a shallow dish, combine the almond flour, grated Parmesan cheese, garlic powder, onion powder, and paprika to make the coating mixture.

3. Dip each cube steak into the beaten eggs, then dredge in the seasoned coating mixture, pressing to adhere.

4. Heat the olive oil (or avocado oil) in a large skillet over medium-high heat.

5. Add the breaded cube steaks to the skillet and cook for 4-5 minutes per side, until golden brown and crispy.

6. Remove the cooked cube steaks from the skillet and transfer to a plate. Cover with foil to keep warm.

7. To make the country gravy, melt the butter in the same skillet over medium heat.

8. Stir in the almond flour to make a roux, cooking for 1-2 minutes until lightly golden.

9. Gradually whisk in the beef broth, stirring constantly to prevent lumps from forming.

10. Continue cooking the gravy until thickened to your desired consistency. Season with salt and pepper to taste.

11. Serve the chicken fried steak hot, topped with the country gravy.

Nutritional value: (per serving)

- Calories: 400

- Protein: 30g

- Fat: 25g

- Carbohydrates: 5g (net carbs)

Keto Meatloaf

Description: This keto meatloaf is a delicious and comforting dish that's perfect for a cozy family dinner. Made with ground beef, almond flour, and a flavorful blend of seasonings, it's a low-carb twist on a classic favorite.

Preparation time: 15 minutes

Cooking time: 1 hour

Ingredients:

- 1 pound ground beef

- 1/2 cup almond flour

- 1/4 cup grated Parmesan cheese

- 1/4 cup tomato sauce or sugar-free ketchup

- 1 egg

- 1 small onion, finely chopped

- 2 cloves garlic, minced

- 1 teaspoon dried oregano

- 1 teaspoon dried basil

- Salt and pepper to taste

- Sugar-free ketchup (optional, for topping)

Directions:

1. Preheat your oven to 350°F (175°C). Grease a loaf pan with cooking spray.

2. In a large mixing bowl, combine the ground beef, almond flour, grated Parmesan cheese,

tomato sauce (or sugar-free ketchup), egg, chopped onion, minced garlic, dried oregano, dried basil, salt, and pepper. Mix until well combined.

3. Transfer the meatloaf mixture to the greased loaf pan, pressing down evenly.

4. If desired, spread a thin layer of sugar-free ketchup over the top of the meatloaf.

5. Bake in the preheated oven for 50-60 minutes, or until the meatloaf is cooked through and the top is golden brown.

6. Remove from the oven and let the meatloaf cool for a few minutes before slicing.

7. Serve hot, accompanied by your favorite low-carb side dishes.

Nutritional value: (per serving, without optional ketchup topping)

- Calories: 300

- Protein: 25g

- Fat: 20g

- Carbohydrates: 5g (net carbs)

Keto Sausage Stuffed Peppers

Description: These keto sausage stuffed peppers are a flavorful and satisfying meal that's perfect for a low-carb lifestyle. Bell peppers stuffed with seasoned sausage and topped with melted cheese make for a delicious and nutritious dinner option.

Preparation time: 15 minutes

Cooking time: 30 minutes

Ingredients:

- 4 bell peppers, halved and seeded

- 1 pound Italian sausage, casings removed

- 1 small onion, diced

- 2 cloves garlic, minced

- 1/2 cup diced tomatoes

- 1/2 cup shredded mozzarella cheese

- Salt and pepper to taste

- Chopped fresh parsley, for garnish (optional)

Directions:

1. Preheat your oven to 375°F (190°C).

2. In a skillet, cook the Italian sausage over medium heat until browned, breaking it apart with a spoon as it cooks.

3. Add the diced onion and minced garlic to the skillet. Cook for 3-4 minutes, until softened.

4. Stir in the diced tomatoes and cook for an additional 2-3 minutes.

5. Season the sausage mixture with salt and pepper to taste.

6. Spoon the sausage mixture evenly into the halved bell peppers, filling each pepper half.

7. Place the stuffed peppers in a baking dish and sprinkle the shredded mozzarella cheese over the top.

8. Bake in the preheated oven for 25-30 minutes, or until the peppers are tender and the cheese is melted and bubbly.

9. Remove from the oven and let cool slightly before serving.

10. Garnish with chopped fresh parsley, if desired.

Nutritional value: (per serving)

- Calories: 350

- Protein: 25g

- Fat: 25g

- Carbohydrates: 8g (net carbs)

Air Fryer Bacon Wrapped Chicken Tenders

Description: These air fryer bacon wrapped chicken tenders are crispy, flavorful, and perfect for a keto-friendly appetizer or main course. Juicy chicken tenders wrapped in crispy bacon make for a delicious and satisfying dish that's sure to be a hit with the whole family.

Preparation time: 10 minutes

Cooking time: 15 minutes

Ingredients:

- 1 pound chicken tenders

- Salt and pepper to taste

- 8 slices bacon

- Toothpicks

Directions:

1. Season the chicken tenders with salt and pepper.

2. Wrap each chicken tender with a slice of bacon, securing the ends with toothpicks.

3. Preheat your air fryer to 400°F (200°C).

4. Place the bacon wrapped chicken tenders in the air fryer basket in a single layer, making sure they are not touching.

5. Cook in the air fryer for 12-15 minutes, flipping halfway through, until the bacon is crispy and the chicken is cooked through.

6. Remove from the air fryer and let cool for a few minutes before serving.

7. Serve hot, accompanied by your favorite dipping sauce.

Nutritional value: (per serving)

- Calories: 300

- Protein: 25g

- Fat: 20g

- Carbohydrates: 0g

Keto Zuppa Toscana Soup

Description: This keto Zuppa Toscana soup is a low-carb version of the classic Olive Garden favorite. Loaded with sausage, bacon, kale, and cauliflower, it's a hearty and comforting soup that's perfect for a cozy night in.

Preparation time: 15 minutes

Cooking time: 30 minutes

Ingredients:

- 1 pound Italian sausage, casings removed

- 6 slices bacon, chopped

- 1 small onion, diced

- 2 cloves garlic, minced

- 4 cups chicken broth

- 1 head cauliflower, chopped into florets

- 2 cups chopped kale

- 1 cup heavy cream

- Salt and pepper to taste

- Grated Parmesan cheese, for serving (optional)

Directions:

1. In a large pot or Dutch oven, cook the Italian sausage and chopped bacon over medium heat until browned, breaking them apart with a spoon as they cook.

2. Add the diced onion and minced garlic to the pot. Cook for 3-4 minutes, until softened.

3. Pour in the chicken broth and bring the mixture to a simmer.

4. Add the chopped cauliflower to the pot and cook for 10-12 minutes, until tender.

5. Stir in the chopped kale and heavy cream. Cook for an additional 5 minutes, until the kale is wilted and the soup is heated through.

6. Season with salt and pepper to taste.

7. Serve hot, garnished with grated Parmesan cheese, if desired.

Nutritional value: (per serving)

- Calories: 350

- Protein: 20g

- Fat: 25g

- Carbohydrates: 7g (net carbs)

Keto Cheeseburger Casserole

Description: This keto cheeseburger casserole is a flavorful and satisfying dish that's perfect for a low-carb dinner. Packed with ground beef, cheese, and all the classic cheeseburger toppings, it's a delicious twist on a family favorite.

Preparation time: 15 minutes

Cooking time: 30 minutes

Ingredients:

- 1 pound ground beef

- 1 small onion, diced

- 2 cloves garlic, minced

- 1/2 cup diced tomatoes

- 1/4 cup sugar-free ketchup

- 1 tablespoon mustard

- 2 cups shredded cheddar cheese

- Salt and pepper to taste

- Chopped pickles, for garnish (optional)

Directions:

1. Preheat your oven to 375°F (190°C). Grease a baking dish with cooking spray.

2. In a skillet, cook the ground beef over medium heat until browned, breaking it apart with a spoon as it cooks.

3. Add the diced onion and minced garlic to the skillet. Cook for 3-4 minutes, until softened.

4. Stir in the diced tomatoes, sugar-free ketchup, and mustard. Cook for an additional 2-3 minutes.

5. Season the ground beef mixture with salt and pepper to taste.

6. Transfer the ground beef mixture to the greased baking dish and spread it out evenly.

7. Sprinkle the shredded cheddar cheese over the top of the ground beef mixture.

8. Bake in the preheated oven for 20-25 minutes, or until the cheese is melted and bubbly.

9. Remove from the oven and let cool slightly before serving.

10. Garnish with chopped pickles, if desired.

Nutritional value: (per serving)

- Calories: 350

- Protein: 25g

- Fat: 25g

- Carbohydrates: 5g (net carbs)

Keto Shrimp Scampi

Description: This keto shrimp scampi is a flavorful and elegant dish that's perfect for a special occasion or a romantic dinner at home. Succulent shrimp cooked in a garlic butter sauce and served over zucchini noodles make for a delicious and low-carb meal option.

Preparation time: 15 minutes

Cooking time: 10 minutes

Ingredients:

- 1 pound shrimp, peeled and deveined

- Salt and pepper to taste

- 4 tablespoons butter

- 4 cloves garlic, minced

- Zest and juice of 1 lemon

- 1/4 cup dry white wine (optional)

- 2 tablespoons chopped fresh parsley

- Zucchini noodles, for serving

Directions:

1. Season the shrimp with salt and pepper.

2. In a large skillet, melt the butter over medium heat. Add the minced garlic and cook for 1 minute, until fragrant.

3. Add the shrimp to the skillet and cook for 2-3 minutes per side, until pink and opaque.

4. Stir in the lemon zest, lemon juice, and dry white wine (if using). Cook for an additional 1-2 minutes.

5. Remove from heat and stir in the chopped fresh parsley.

6. Serve the shrimp scampi hot, spooned over zucchini noodles.

    Nutritional value: (per serving, without zucchini noodles)

- Calories: 250

- Protein: 25g

- Fat: 15g

- Carbohydrates: 3g (net carbs)

Chapter 8

Snacking the Carnivore Way

Beef Jerky

Description: Beef jerky is a savory, protein-packed snack made from thinly sliced beef that's been seasoned and dried to preserve it. It's perfect for on-the-go snacking or as a protein boost during outdoor activities.

Preparation time: 20 minutes (plus marinating time)

Cooking time: 3-6 hours

Ingredients:

- 1 pound of lean beef (such as flank steak or round steak), thinly sliced

- ¼ cup soy sauce

- 2 tablespoons Worcestershire sauce

- 2 teaspoons smoked paprika

- 1 teaspoon garlic powder

- 1 teaspoon onion powder

- ½ teaspoon black pepper

- Optional: red pepper flakes for heat

Directions:

1. In a bowl, mix together soy sauce, Worcestershire sauce, smoked paprika, garlic powder, onion powder, black pepper, and red pepper flakes if desired.

2. Add the thinly sliced beef to the marinade, ensuring each piece is coated evenly. Cover the bowl and refrigerate for at least 4 hours, or preferably overnight, to allow the flavors to penetrate the meat.

3. Preheat your oven to 175°F (80°C) or the lowest setting available.

4. Remove the beef from the marinade and pat it dry with paper towels to remove excess moisture.

5. Arrange the beef slices on a wire rack set over a baking sheet, ensuring they are not touching each other.

6. Place the baking sheet in the oven and bake for 3-6 hours, or until the beef is dry and leathery.

The exact time will depend on the thickness of your slices and your oven's temperature.

7. Once the beef jerky is done, let it cool completely before storing in an airtight container or resealable bags.

   Nutritional value: Beef jerky is a high-protein snack, typically low in fat and carbohydrates. It provides essential nutrients like iron, zinc, and B vitamins. However, commercial varieties may contain added sodium and preservatives, so homemade versions allow for better control over ingredients.

Pepperoni Slices

Description: Pepperoni slices are a classic topping for pizzas, sandwiches, and appetizers. Making your own allows you to control the quality of ingredients and customize the flavor to your preference.

Preparation time: 15 minutes

Cooking time: 2-3 hours

Ingredients:

- 1 pound of ground pork or beef

- 1 tablespoon paprika

- 1 teaspoon garlic powder

- 1 teaspoon onion powder

- 1 teaspoon dried oregano

- 1 teaspoon fennel seeds

- ½ teaspoon cayenne pepper (adjust to taste)

- Salt and black pepper to taste

Directions:

1. In a bowl, combine ground pork or beef with paprika, garlic powder, onion powder, dried oregano, fennel seeds, cayenne pepper, salt, and black pepper. Mix until well combined.

2. Divide the mixture in half and shape each portion into a log.

3. Wrap each log tightly in plastic wrap and refrigerate for at least 1 hour to firm up.

4. Preheat your oven to 200°F (95°C).

5. Unwrap the chilled logs and slice them thinly using a sharp knife or a meat slicer.

6. Arrange the pepperoni slices on a baking sheet lined with parchment paper, ensuring they are not touching.

7. Bake in the preheated oven for 2-3 hours, or until the pepperoni slices are crispy and slightly browned.

8. Remove from the oven and let them cool completely before using or storing in an airtight container.

Nutritional value: Homemade pepperoni slices can be a good source of protein and essential nutrients like iron and zinc. However, their nutritional value may vary based on the type of meat used and any added ingredients.

Hard-Boiled Eggs

Description: Hard-boiled eggs are a versatile and nutritious snack or ingredient in many dishes. They are easy to prepare and can be enjoyed on their own, sliced in salads, or as a protein-rich addition to meals.

Preparation time: 5 minutes

Cooking time: 10-12 minutes

Ingredients:

- Eggs (as many as desired)

Directions:

1. Place the eggs in a single layer in a saucepan or pot.

2. Add enough water to cover the eggs by at least 1 inch.

3. Bring the water to a boil over medium-high heat.

4. Once the water reaches a rolling boil, cover the saucepan with a lid and remove it from the heat.

5. Let the eggs sit in the hot water for 10-12 minutes for hard-boiled eggs.

6. While the eggs are cooking, prepare a bowl of ice water.

7. After the cooking time is up, carefully remove the eggs from the hot water and place them in the ice water bath to cool rapidly and stop the cooking process.

8. Let the eggs cool in the ice water for a few minutes.

9. Once cooled, gently tap each egg on a hard surface to crack the shell, then peel away the shell.

10. Rinse the peeled eggs under cold water to remove any remaining shell fragments.

11. Hard-boiled eggs can be stored in the refrigerator for up to one week.

Nutritional value: Hard-boiled eggs are rich in protein, vitamins, and minerals, including vitamin D, vitamin B12, selenium, and choline. They are low in calories and can contribute to feelings of fullness and satisfaction.

Pork Rinds

Description: Pork rinds, also known as chicharrones, are crispy fried pork skin snacks popular in many cuisines. They are crunchy, savory, and often seasoned with spices for extra flavor.

Preparation time: 5 minutes

Cooking time: 30-40 minutes

Ingredients:

- Pork skin with fat attached

- Salt and spices (optional)

Directions:

1. Preheat your oven to 325°F (160°C).

2. Rinse the pork skin under cold water and pat it dry with paper towels.

3. Cut the pork skin into small pieces, about 1-2 inches in size.

4. Arrange the pork skin pieces in a single layer on a baking sheet lined with parchment paper.

5. Sprinkle the pork skin with salt and any desired spices or seasonings.

6. Place the baking sheet in the preheated oven and bake for 30-40 minutes, or until the pork rinds are crispy and golden brown.

7. Remove the pork rinds from the oven and let them cool slightly before serving.

8. Enjoy pork rinds as a crunchy snack or use them as a topping for salads, soups, or other dishes.

Nutritional value: Pork rinds are high in protein and fat, making them a satisfying snack option. However, they are also high in calories and sodium, so they should be enjoyed in moderation as part of a balanced diet.

Salmon or Tuna Pouches

Description: Salmon or tuna pouches are convenient and portable options for enjoying canned fish. They're great for quick meals, snacks, or adding protein to salads and sandwiches.

Preparation time: 5 minutes

Cooking time: None

Ingredients:

- Canned salmon or tuna

- Optional seasonings (such as lemon juice, olive oil, herbs, or spices)

Directions:

1. Open the pouch of canned salmon or tuna.

2. Drain any excess liquid from the pouch.

3. Transfer the salmon or tuna to a bowl.

4. If desired, add seasonings such as lemon juice, olive oil, herbs, or spices to taste.

5. Mix well to combine the seasonings with the fish.

6. Serve the salmon or tuna straight from the pouch or use it in your favorite recipes.

Nutritional value: Salmon and tuna are excellent sources of protein and omega-3 fatty acids, which are beneficial for heart health and brain function. They also provide essential nutrients like vitamin D and selenium. However, be mindful of added sodium in canned varieties, and choose options packed in water or olive oil for healthier choices.

Conclusion

As we come to the end of our journey through the world of the Carnivore Diet, it's time to reflect on the transformative power of this remarkable lifestyle and the profound impact it can have on our health, well-being, and overall quality of life. Throughout the pages of this book, we've explored the depths of carnivore living, from its evolutionary origins to its modern-day resurgence as a potent tool for reclaiming our health and vitality. We've delved into the science behind the diet, unraveling its nutritional foundations and dispelling myths and misconceptions along the way. We've provided you with practical guidance and support to help you succeed on your carnivore journey, from stocking your kitchen with the essentials to navigating social situations with confidence and grace. And we've shared with you a treasure trove of tantalizing recipes, each one crafted to showcase the diverse flavors and textures of the carnivore diet.

But beyond the practicalities of meal planning and food preparation, the Carnivore Diet is ultimately about reclaiming our birthright as human beings—rediscovering the simple joy of nourishing our bodies with the foods that nature intended. It's about reconnecting with our primal instincts, honoring the wisdom of our ancestors, and embracing the innate intelligence of our bodies to guide us toward optimal health and well-being. And it's about recognizing that true health is not just the absence of disease, but a state of vitality, energy, and vitality that allows us to thrive in every aspect of our lives.

As you embark on your own carnivore journey, remember that you are not alone. You are part of a vibrant and growing community of individuals who have dared to challenge the status quo, who have refused to accept mediocrity, and who have embraced the transformative power of the carnivore lifestyle. Draw strength from their stories, their successes, and their unwavering commitment to reclaiming their health and vitality. And know that you have everything you need to succeed within you—the wisdom, the courage, and the determination to create the life you deserve.

So as you close the pages of this book and step out into the world, remember that the journey is just beginning. Embrace the challenges that lie ahead, celebrate the victories, and never lose sight of the incredible potential that lies within you. And above all, trust in the wisdom of your body, for it knows better than anyone what it needs to thrive. With each bite you take, each meal you savor, and each day you live as a carnivore, you'll be one step closer to unlocking the boundless potential that awaits you on this extraordinary journey. So go forth with courage, with confidence, and with a sense of adventure, and may your carnivore journey be filled with health, happiness, and endless possibilities.